The Myeloma Survival Guide

Essential Advice For Patients And Their Loved Ones

Jim Tamkin, MD
Dave Visel

16
EasyRead Large

RHYW

Copyright Page from the Original Book

Visit our website at www.demoshealth.com

ISBN: 978-1-936303-68-7
e-book ISBN: 978-1-617052-24-8

Acquisitions Editor: Julia Pastore
Compositor: diacriTech, Chennai, India

Medical information provided by Demos Health, in the absence of a visit with a health care professional, must be considered as an educational service only. This book is not designed to replace a physician's independent judgment about the appropriateness or risks of a procedure or therapy for a given patient. Our purpose is to provide you with information that will help you make your own health care decisions.

The information and opinions provided here are believed to be accurate and sound, based on the best judgment available to the authors, editors, and publisher, but readers who fail to consult appropriate health authorities assume the risk of injuries. The publisher is not responsible for errors or omissions. The editors and publisher welcome any reader to report to the publisher any discrepancies or inaccuracies noticed.

Library of Congress Cataloging-in-Publication Data

Tamkin, James A., author.
The myeloma survival guide: essential advice for patients and their loved ones / Jim Tamkin, MD and Dave Visel.
pages cm
Includes bibliographical references and index.
ISBN 978-1-936303-68-7 (alk. paper)—ISBN 978-1-61705-224-8 (e-book)
1. Multiple myeloma. 2. Multiple myeloma—Treatment. I. Visel, Dave, author. II. Title.
RC280.B6T35 2013
616.99'418—dc23
2014003153

Printed in the United States of America by McNaughton & Gunn.
14 15 16 17 18 / 5 4 3 2 1

TABLE OF CONTENTS

Praise for The Myeloma Survival Guide

"Dr. Jim Tamkin has turned his own illness into a benefit for patients with myeloma worldwide. Together with Dave Visel, they have developed a literal GPS system, an invaluable guide to patients with newly diagnosed multiple myeloma. Not only have they provided clear information on the disease and its treatment, but most importantly also convey critical guidance on how to deal with the very personal life-impacting effects of this disease for patients and family members alike. In this era of great excitement in myeloma where novel therapies are changing the treatment paradigm and improving patient outcome, this book assures awareness and access to patients and caregivers of these advances, so that patients can enjoy longer and higher quality lives with their loved ones. There simply is no greater gift than this."

Kenneth C. Anderson, MD
Kraft Family Professor of Medicine, Harvard Medical School
Chief, Division of Hematologic Neoplasia
Director, Jerome Lipper Multiple Myeloma Center and LeBow Institute for Myeloma Therapeutics
Dana-Farber Cancer Institute
Boston, Massachusetts

"*The Myeloma Survival Guide* is filled with facts, factoids, tidbits, and anecdotal descriptions that would help anyone starting on their myeloma adventure. We have come a long way since the advent of transplants with the discovery of new novel agents and the combination therapies. There is much to learn and much to do. I was pleased that Dr. Tamkin takes into account the vast differences in approach to the disease, its treatment and whether or not cure is real. I would definitely recommend the book to my patients and their caregivers."

Bart Barlogie, MD, PhD
Director, Myeloma Institute for Research and Therapy
Winthrop Rockefeller Cancer Institute
University of Arkansas

"It's tremendous for new patients to have this book. A myeloma diagnosis is overwhelming. Even as a physician, I did almost nothing but read for a month after my myeloma was confirmed. One of this book's greatest values is that it covers everything in one place."

Burton Dickey, MD
Myeloma Patient
Professor and Chair, Department of Pulmonary Medicine
MD Anderson Cancer Center
Houston, Texas

"This is the ultimate guide for all patients and caregivers as they navigate through the rapidly changing landscape of the myeloma diagnosis and treatment process. The authors have poignantly written *The Myeloma Survival Guide* from the unique perspectives of the patient and caregiver. The intimate knowledge of living with cancer allowed the authors to highlight common health and psychosocial concerns as patients are living longer than ever."

Beth Faiman, PhDc, MSN, APN-BC
Multiple Myeloma Nurse Practitioner
Taussig Cancer Institute
Cleveland Clinic
Cleveland, Ohio

"This is a wonderful primer for myeloma patients and their caregivers. It provides up to date knowledge while at the same time providing practical pointers for patients and caregivers to deal with this horrible disease. Since knowledge is power, this book will provide essential tools to allow patients and caregivers weather the 'myeloma storm' more prepared. I wholeheartedly recommend it."

Sergio A. Giralt, MD
Chief, Adult Bone Marrow Transplant Service
Memorial Sloan-Kettering Cancer Center
New York City

"As a patient, I understand how difficult it is for patients and their families to manage the uncertainties of a multiple myeloma diagnosis. Dave Visel and Dr. Jim Tamkin have collaborated to develop a detailed resource for approaching this situation, which will undoubtedly help newly diagnosed myeloma patients and their caregivers attain the information that they need to empower themselves throughout their journey with myeloma."

Kathy Giusti
Founder and CEO
Multiple Myeloma Research Foundation

"This book is very good! It is direct and comprehensive and features just about anything and everything new myeloma patients, caregivers and family members need to know."

Pat Killingsworth
Multiple Myeloma Patient
Medical Journalist and Freelance Medical Writer

"I will hand this book to new myeloma patients, knowing that it will give them tools and a confidence that they would not have gotten without it. The teaching is clear, complete, accurate, easy to follow, memorable, and occasionally very funny. It produces better prepared patients for their oncologists to treat. When I learned that I had myeloma in 2007, I looked for this book. It was not there. Even though I had access to the medical faculty of a great university, my pathway to survival followed a much tougher road than you will be shown here. If you are a myeloma patient, or a caregiver, the key to the future is in your hands. Don't put it down."

John W. Killip, DDS
Myeloma Patient
Clinical Professor Emeritus
University of Missouri School of Dentistry
Kansas City, Missouri

"We have needed this authoritative, comprehensive, encouraging reinforcement for myeloma patients for at least ten years. A copy should be placed in the hands of every new myeloma patient at the time of diagnosis."

Robert A. Kyle, MD
Professor of Medicine, Laboratory Medicine and Pathology
Mayo Clinic Cancer Center
Rochester, Minnesota

"In a word, it's *fabulous!* I can find nothing lacking in style or substance in this treatise on myeloma. I have been studying the literature on myeloma since my diagnosis in 2006. I have interviewed eight different doctors (five oncologists) relative to my treatment. Almost all of what I've discovered is in the first 90 pages and I've still got some reading to do! I've received written 'what to expect' documents from both the City of Hope and the Veteran's Administration—neither of which is this complete, enlightening or well written. The authors have produced a well-documented ... [and] wonderful tool for oncologists treating myeloma and their patients, caregivers and other interested parties."

Duke Rohlffs
Myeloma Patient
Mesquite, Nevada

Also by Dave Visel
Living with Cancer: A Practical Guide

Also by Jim Tamkin
Manual of Ambulatory Medicine
(with Alan S. Robbins, MD)

We wish to thank the Vasek and Anna Maria Polak Charitable Foundation and its Director, Soterios F. Menzelos, for the wise counsel and generous financial support that underpinned this project from its inception.

Preface

Hang in and hold on.

You've been mugged. They didn't steal your wallet. They stole your life. And there's nobody you can call to get it back.

You did nothing wrong. At least nothing either you or the medical world can figure out. Your number just came up.

Multiply the U.S. population times. 0000625. That's your number.

Thought of another way, your disease strikes one in 16,000.

You could have won a lottery beating odds like that. Instead you're stuck with an incurable disease called myeloma.

Myeloma. As a name, it doesn't even have the decency to be catchy.

Or famous. Nobody's heard of it. When you tell people what's wrong with you, they say, "Huh?"

That's what you said when the doc first introduced it to you, isn't it?

The other thing that's really irritating is the unpredictability. There are at least half a dozen different ways myeloma can make you sick or bring you pain or give you some weird side effect like double vision or numb hands or back pain. It chooses one or all of them without warning. You shuttle from doctor to doctor for help. Sometimes it's worth it. Sometimes not.

I'm pretty sure that the moment of your diagnosis was unlike any experience before or since. When you heard, *I'm terribly sorry to tell you ...* the shock hit like a ton of bricks. You felt like you'd fallen into a dark, lonely place with nothing but questions and fears. Abandoned. Vulnerable.

I call it *no man's land.*

If you haven't realized it yet, please know that soon, out of this confusion, darkness and fear, sanity will reappear. Yes, you have cancer. Yes, the situation is bad. But you have company. There are lifeguards on duty and ways for you to get to safety.

All sorts of help is coming, including people who intend to do things for you that you didn't know needed doing and won't be thrilled about.

Over 80,000 Americans – like me – have been plunged into this awful illness ahead of you and are still here. A lot's going on in research. We've benefited, and so will you.

This sharing of life with an obscure incurable illness is no five-star accommodation. But the assembled experts in these pages offer you the best available ways to maximize damage control and—perhaps—to extend life.

Hang in and hold on.

Jim Tamkin, MD

Introduction

This is the myeloma patient's guide to survival.

While a cure is yet to come, it may not be necessary. Several avenues to prolonged, high quality coexistence with this cancer are being demonstrated and continuously improved.

With proper disease management, over 120,000 myeloma patients, who would have died, will credit normal or near normal lives to recent events in the few years just ahead.

How Come Nobody's Heard of Myeloma?

In a world of practical limitations, the cancers that attack millions receive far more attention than the cancers that attack thousands. Out of a total U.S. annual expenditure of $280 billion for cancer treatment and research in 2012, a pittance went into fighting myeloma and other rare afflictions.

Nobody's marching for myeloma. There's no symbol that everyone recognizes.

Many confuse it with melanoma, a dangerous but wholly unrelated skin cancer.

Meanwhile, dramatic medical progress is being made. This is a new day for both myeloma patients and their physicians.

Background

In 1845, a patient with excruciating broken-bone-like pain and heat-soluble animal matter in the urine was studied. The disease responsible came to be known as multiple myeloma because of tumors spreading through the bones of legs, pelvis, back and skull. Though treatments to ease pain and to slow its advance have been developed over the past 150 years, no definitive cause is known, or cure.

European cultures experience moderate rates of the disease while black descendents of African races are two to three times more likely to be afflicted. Asians suffer it least often. Statistics for Native Americans are unreliable. We also know that 60% of its victims will be men and that it usually emerges in mid to late life. A usually harmless condition called monoclonal gammopathy of undetermined significance (MGUS) always occurs first. About three percent of those with MGUS, as it is universally known, eventually get myeloma. How either disease selects those it strikes or why others escape them are also mysteries.

Whatever ethnicity or age—or length of time with MGUS—death usually followed the onset of myeloma within two or three years, until recently.

How This Book Was Written

Jim Tamkin, MD, FACP, FACE, a Los Angeles internist and endocrinologist, was diagnosed with multiple myeloma in 1999. At the time, life expectancy after the appearance of the cancer averaged 33 months.

Shortly thereafter, Dr. Tamkin visited the five leading myeloma oncologists in the United States and adopted a therapy program based on a composite of their recommendations. Though his disease remained aggressive, he was able to successfully manage it through a series of innovative chemotherapy protocols, until a sudden turn for the worse in December 2010, 11 years after diagnosis.

Dave Visel met and interviewed Dr. Tamkin in 2001 as part of another book Visel was writing, *Living with Cancer.* Their meetings were candid and intense, with neither expecting to see the other again—at least not in this world.

So it was a pleasant surprise for them to meet again in March 2009. They discussed 'Tamkin's survival at length, realizing that what was coming to be known about managing this still incurable disease would be of great importance to new myeloma patients.

The next 18 months were given to co-development of this project. Though Dr. Tamkin died in March 2011, the amount of time he had focused on myeloma therapies and disease management strategies may exceed that of anyone else in the world.

A general book outline, interviews, points of view, voluminous notes and several chapters were in place before Dr. Tamkin's passing, which Visel finished in the name of the partnership

In addition, well over a hundred other distinguished men and women of medicine, other sciences, the law, education, health insurance, and public service have contributed their expertise to this book.

Earnings

All of the authors' earnings from the sale of this book go to the TBA Foundation, a nonprofit charity that Dr. Tamkin and Mr. Visel founded in 2009.

Part One

First Steps

1

Take Charge: You Don’t Get to Just Sit There

Supervise your case.

The Nut of It

Your health care team wants you to understand the situation. It knows that if you do understand, and if you actively participate in the discussion of your treatment program, you will be a more successful patient.

Can I Do This?

So here you are. Not feeling your best. Angry. Scared. Being presented with scientific jargon (see the Glossary for myeloma-specific explanations of the words and terms you don’t understand) and machines and decisions that would confound a PhD—and you've just started reading a chapter that says that this is *your* ship to steer.

The situation is actually worse than that. Research indicates that more than half of those who get multiple myeloma don't know what's happening or why. The result for them is catastrophic.

This is not just a ship—it is a ship in crisis. You are not just steering, you are directing both boat and crew. Your sailors are reporting awful things like boiler room failure and holes in the hull. They are recommending which to fix, and how—to you.

Decide to step up to this task and, together, we will make sure that you succeed.

Use It or Lose It

"I was a mile into my treadmill workout when coverage began to air of a healthcare forum at the White House. As I watched, I found myself gradually gaining speed, growing more and more upset."

At this point in her essay published in the *Los Angeles Times,* Valerie Ulene, MD, a preventive medicine specialist, reveals a long-simmering frustration: "The plan demanded fundamental change from insurance companies, hospitals, and healthcare providers, and failed to address what patients have to do."

We aren't holding people accountable for their unhealthful behaviors, she says. Particularly after you discover that you have a serious illness, you must take care of yourself. If you don't know what to do—and no one does on day 1—find out. Then take responsibility for getting the tests, seeing the specialists, doing the fact-finding, and reorganizing your life; whatever is necessary. is necessary.

Find out what to do—that's why this book is open before you—and get'er done.

Your Take-charge Tools:

- Don't expect the government or anybody else to run this treatment program for you.
- Don't do it alone. Get a partner–caregiver.
- See the Glossary in the back of this book for definitions of myeloma-specific terms.
- Keep good records.
- Know the goal you are working toward.

First Thing: Get a Partner–Caregiver

As a myeloma patient, you are beginning a long, complicated, physically and mentally taxing journey. There will be doctors and insurance people and hospital and lab people—also bankers and lawyers and your friends to deal with. On top of that, all the demands and responsibilities you had before you got sick are still there.

You may think you can handle this mess by yourself. Don't try it. You will screw up in ways that you will deeply regret. Get someone by your side, helping you keep your house in order.

Everybody needs somebody. The Lone Ranger had Tonto. DeBakey had Ochsner.

Partner–Caregiver Candidates

If you are married, consider reading this chapter and the next two with your spouse beside you. Think about the pros and cons of using your marriage partnership as the springboard for caregiving. There are a dozen reasons why a spouse should take on this job. There may be strong arguments against it. Only the two of you can sort this matter out.

Next option: Recruit another family member or a friend. This sort of team often works well, even if this person has no qualifications beyond friendship and a willingness to try.

Before exploring this choice, be warned that yours will become a very personal relationship. You will need somebody with maturity and staying power.

You may also elect to hire a professional caregiver. While paid help is financially draining, a person who knows how to give a shot, has a driver's license, and is strong enough to help you get about may be a wise investment.

A variation on this theme is to reserve paid assistance for the times that you and your partner–caregiver need peaking power.

Caregivers Not to Hire

If you employ a paid helper, look for daily evidence that your caregiver cares about you. You will see plenty of the other kind helping the halt and the lame in the offices of the doctors you visit. These obviously bored help mates, providing dissolute service, make thoughtless, dangerous mistakes.

Even if you hire a personal nurse from one of the medical concierge services that prowl high-rent districts, be certain that you have put yourself into enthusiastic helping hands.

A candidate caregiver who comes out of the hospice industry may not be a good choice. We will all approach that *great gettin' up morning* one day. Let's not make it a day next week. Work with someone who thinks more about remission and your bucket *list* than about the kicking of the darn thing.

Keep Thorough, Well-Organized Treatment Records

One of the benefits of being in charge is that you will make a point of noticing what's going on in the offices and laboratories you visit.

Illness and Treatment History
(From the date myeloma was discovered to the present)

Name: ______
Year: ______

Date	Condition	Physician	Treatment
1/3/14	Fell. May have fractured a rib.	Jane Doe, MD, our long-time family doctor	X-ray revealed
1/6/14	Fracture and other conditions need to be diagnosed.	Dr. Doe	Ribs taped. Blood samples taken. MRI.

Each keeps its own records. Some are scanty. Some are so voluminous that details are hard to find. None includes all the records from all the other places you go for help. You are the tie that binds.

Illnesses and Treatments

A simple history including date, the reason you went to the doctor, the doctor's name and specialty, and medical tests and treatments, could look like this:

This simple table can be created with a pencil and ruler on notepaper. If you have access to a computer, a table like this one can be created in Word, in Excel, or in any of many other programs. Keep the information short, legible, and current. Be careful to spell medical terminology accurately.

> "I have found that since I began keeping careful records of my treatments and side effects, I have better conversations with my doctor."
>
> *—Doug B.*

Drugs, Herbs, Vitamins, and Supplements

You should also carry a record of all of your drugs, herbs, vitamins, and supplements: name, size of the dose (often in "mg" or milligrams), and how frequently you take it. Keep the list current and simple. Do not forget to include any chemotherapy drugs, blood infusions, or other serum product. List any allergies and allergic reactions or side effects you experience.

These data will help many of the healers you visit. It is also a safety measure. *Oh, you've taken dexamethasone. Then we should...*

Sample:

Date	Medication	Dosage (mg)	Frequency	Notes

Date	Vitamins/Herbs/Supplements	Dosage	Frequency

Blank forms suitable for both an illness history and a current medication record can be found at www.tbafoundation.org/forms.html

Prescriptions, Receipts, and Test Results

You will also need file folders to keep all of your prescriptions, receipts, and test results. If you're told to do or get something, get a prescription or written order. Try to never leave the office of someone who has told you to get something without the prescription for it. Always keep a copy of the prescription in your files.

Also save phone numbers, addresses, patient ID numbers, and names of key contacts.

Myeloma Manager Software

If you or your partner is computer savvy, the International Myeloma Foundation sponsored the creation of disease management software, *Myeloma Manager, Personal Care Assistant,* which is offered as a free download at its website, www.myeloma.org. It is thorough and myeloma-treatment specific. It is easy to use. However, entries must be made almost daily, which can make it become an insistent chore. Some find that keeping file folders and maybe a three-ring binder are a sufficient alternative.

Either way, you will be quickly lost if you don't establish a good record keeping system and maintain it.

Long-Range Goals

One cannot leave a discussion of taking charge without deciding, *Of what?* What are your goals?

The physicians treating your disease seem to have one of two objectives in mind for you. Some want to find a cure. Others will guide you into any port that shelters you from the present storm.

"I think the focus on curing myeloma has been distracting for both my colleagues and their patients," says Sergio A. Giralt, MD, Chief, Adult Bone Marrow Transplant Service, Memorial Sloan-Kettering Cancer Center, New York City. Patients do a lot better when treatment decisions are based on a balance of estimations.

First, patient and medical team should look at how a proposed new treatment may affect patient longevity, then at how it may affect quality of life.

If these two questions seem simple to you, reconsider. Each can be multilayered and quite complex. Each deserves input from your myeloma specialists.

If the answers for longevity and life quality encourage it, evaluate how burdensome the treatment will be for you; exactly how, from the patient's point of view. Is it worth it? What are you buying? What are you giving up?

Some medical procedures may only be effective once. Others can only be effective if your kidney health or some other specific condition meets criteria that could change. Is this the time to chamber your silver bullet?

Dr. Giralt explains that treatment innovations and drug developments have brought us into an era in which many myeloma patients will outlive current four-or five-year estimations—may be by decades. Though probably not cured, their disease will be controlled, become indolent—detectable but not aggressive—or go into remission, no longer detectable.

The goal of Dr. Giralt's treatment strategy is a tie, not a win. Given the finality of losing, and the so far unsuccessful search for a cure, it is a third alternative to seriously consider.

If you adopt this goal, you should share it with your caregiver, family, and friends. Your selection of a medical team will be influenced. There are treatments and clinics your goal will steer you toward and others you will be directed away from.

When You Hear Hoof Beats, Think Horses Not Zebras

The worst thing about being in charge is that you have to accept responsibility for what's decided. Here are a few rules for the decision maker's road:

- When diagnosing, first consider the obvious. (Sutton's Law[1])
- Does it pass the giggle test? (Can you seriously consider the idea?)
- Sometimes the hardest thing in life is to know which bridge to cross and which to burn. (Eric Warren Singer)
- To know little and to be proud of knowing little is disrespectful. (Peggy Noonan)
- Battles are fought by scared men who'd rather be someplace else. (James Bassett)
- Any fool can make a rule, and any fool will mind it. (Henry David Thoreau)

---

1 Not Dr. Sutton; Willie Sutton, the Chicago gangster; for example, Why do you rob banks? Because that's where the money is.

2

Today's To-Do List: Easy, Important Next Steps

Get organized.

Recognize that You are a Changed Person

You are not the same person you were before multiple myeloma. You cannot ever be that premyeloma person again. Insist that others recognize the new you as well. No pretends. No if-onlys. Don't whisper myeloma's name or give it some cutesy-pie nickname. You've got what you've got. Now's the time to do something about it.

Geraldine Ferraro lost her battle with myeloma on March 24, 2011, but her contributions to disease management and the attention she directed toward this disease in Washington, D.C. were gifts to you.

After her diagnosis in the fall of 1998, at age 63, Ferraro's priorities changed. Her law firm partnership, her three-term congressional clout, the prestige of having been the first female vice presidential nominee of a major party and doyen of the D.C. circuit, lost their priorities. Her husband, children, and grandchildren became her focus and in turn they became a team intent on supporting her.

"Your perspective is different when you're walking around with cancer," Ferraro said.

The day of her diagnosis, her husband of many years, John Zaccaro, became her dedicated caregiver in the fight. "John is always by my side," she acknowledged. "He listens. He takes the notes in treatment conferences. He looks up the studies and the new terms, makes follow-up phone calls, sends e-mails."

Laura, youngest daughter and a pediatrician, tracked her mom's progress at a physician's level, cross-examining medical staff and her parents.

John Jr., the middle child and an MBA, managed Zaccaro's businesses, freeing his dad to do whatever was necessary for his mom.

Donna, the eldest, an MBA with a background in television production, helped run the political and public side of her | mother's life.

Each member of the family became engaged and helped using their unique gifts and talents.

Seven years into the fight, Madeleine Albright, former Secretary of State and an equally alpha female, called on the occasion of Ferraro's 70th birthday. "Madeleine, I'm bald, at the beach, recuperating from a stem cell transplant," Ferraro told her. "I'm doing great..."

Ferraro had wound down her law practice, ramped up time for grandchildren, improved her golf swing, started writing a book on aging, and had become an effective advocate for better health care legislation. She was responsible for the Geraldine Ferraro Blood Cancer Education Program, now a part of the National Institutes of Health.

She was also a myeloma soul mate. People phoned her. She phoned them. She became famous for myeloma talks in supermarket checkout lines and anywhere the topic came up. She counseled Senator Kay Bailey Hutchinson when the senator's brother was diagnosed. She became a friend and supporter of Kathy Giusti, head of the Multiple Myeloma Research Foundation, who was also a long-surviving myeloma patient.

Ferraro realized that her life had changed and immediately changed her life. She recognized the dangers of her disease and mobilized, accepting the support of others and offering support in return. Her approach may be a useful example for you.

> It is very helpful to involve your caregiver in every decision and activity related to the new you.

Get a Guru

The leader of your treatment team must be a medical doctor (MD or DO):

- whose specialty is cancer (oncology),
- who is an expert in blood diseases (hematology), and
- who has treated other multiple myeloma patients.

The doctor who diagnosed you may have these qualifications. If not, he or she may already be looking for this specialist for you. Your disease is rare and commonly misunderstood. The latest treatment regimen has not been used by that many folks.

A referral within the medical community—doctor-to-doctor—is the most likely way you are going to get into the right hands. If you live in or near a city, there's a good chance that the diagnosing doctor can do this for you.

If that doesn't work, pick a cancer treatment center specializing in myeloma. Contact it and let the institution assign you the expert you need from its staff. Be open to travel.

A list of hospitals with notable myeloma treatment and disease management teams is at the end of this chapter.

Go with the Flow

Visits and tests will lead to more visits and tests. Your guru, or the hospital you chose, will cause other professional specialties to come to your aid. The treatment team for a myeloma patient will build to half a dozen doctors plus technicians and nurses in no time. Don't get in the way of this process. Let it happen. Watch and learn how to work with each specialty.

Separate the Sheep from the Goats

As this team-building is taking place, friends, family, and others will be interested. Some of them will have medicinal suggestions they *know* will help you. Stop and ponder this interesting phenomenon: Why would someone who has absolutely no experience dealing with this rare, complicated, dangerous disease prescribe for you? Vitamin Q. Lionized water. African anthill dirt. Some mystery substance sold out of an online pharmacy in Uzbekistan.

Really?

Be nice to these people. They want to help. Had they thought about it, they might have realized that they are endangering your well-being. But they never do. This urge to prescribe is a curious part of the times in which we live; probably the result of too many hospital shows on television.

If Auntie Em's home remedy seems compelling, discuss it with your guru. Some traditional or folk remedies make people feel better and if they don't get in the way of the high-octane tools your medical team counts on, your docs won't care if you use them.

Be warned that sometimes these bromides clash with your mainline drugs. Sometimes seriously. Examples:

- Green tea and Velcade
- Iron supplements and Aredia or Zometa

Work on Your Elevator Speech

Years ago, some salesman came up with the idea that the most effective explanation for anything should require no more time than it takes for you and the listener to rise one floor in an elevator.

You need a simple, truthful explanation of what's wrong with you. It should include the name of your cancer—call it either myeloma or multiple myeloma. Something to explain it like, *a cancer in my bones.* There will be those who want more details. They will ask questions. You can expound.

Children and senior citizens may need something less brutally frank. Your doc has faced this question before and should have a good suggestion for the situations you expect to face.

Myeloma is frequently confused with melanoma, a nasty skin cancer. If you later hear that people think you have skin cancer, that is probably where the misunderstanding started.

Get Your Health Insurance Coverage Started

Chapter 6 covers this in detail, with very specific instructions. Read it soon.

> **Don't have health insurance?**
>
> Provisions of the Affordable Care Act make it easy to get full coverage. But myeloma-related expenses during the first six months that your new insurance is in effect may not be covered. A little background and some pointers are in Chapter 6.

Have You Gotten a Qualified, Independent Second Opinion of What's Wrong with You?

In all of the nation's leading hospitals, a diagnosis of multiple myeloma is automatically reviewed by the *tumor board,* a panel of highly qualified physicians that meets regularly. If the opinions of that panel of experts leads to any worry that your diagnosis could be incorrect, your case is re-examined. This is a careful system, designed by experienced people with your welfare as the first and foremost concern.

If you were not diagnosed in a major hospital, your finding may not have been reviewed by a second expert. You should check. If this verification step has not been taken, you should ensure that an independent second opinion of your case is obtained right away.

If the second opinion does not agree with the first, get a third.

We know that our doctors have devoted their lives to caring for us, so it seems insulting to demand multiple opinions. No less an authority than the American Society of Clinical Oncology strongly recommends second opinions for all myeloma patients, as will your insurance company.

Need help knowing how to go about getting a second opinion? Call the Bloch Cancer Foundation, 800-433-0464, or visit www.BlochCenter.org.

Prayer

If prayer is an active part of your life you can move on to item number 9 on the To-Do List. But if you are inclined to skepticism of *the God thing,* give us another 30 seconds here.

When W.C. Fields was dying of cancer at an Encino, California, rest home, a visitor found him reading a Bible. "Bill, you're an atheist. What are you doing?"

"Looking for loopholes," the great comic replied.

Struggling by yourself with either the Christian or Jewish Bible, notoriously hard reads, isn't necessary.

Consider returning to a place of worship you once visited. If you drop the slightest hint of interest, your medical team will produce a chaplain. Call a friend you know who has active religious ties.

More than 1,200 scientific studies in the United States since 1975 have focused on the therapeutic effects of active worship, according to Dwight L. Carlson, MD, prominent psychiatrist and best-selling author. More than 800 of them documented a positive result.

Science has certified that an active relationship with the God of your understanding is an effective cancer fighter.

Tell Everyone Who Needs to Know that You Have Myeloma

Your objective is clear, basic information. The telling may be tough. Some anger or tears may come into it. Excessive drama could follow.

They all know that cancer is life-threatening. Kids and the feeble-minded may ask when you are going to die. Other questions, from the intimate to the outrageous, will come at you. They hurt less if you smile and give loving, positive answers.

Think about what to tell each one, and why. Think about the impact of your words. Imagine how the words you use may be misconstrued as one person tells the next.

- You do not want someone screeching into your driveway, hysterical, having heard that you are at death's door.
- You do not want someone to whom you owe money initiating a collection action because of the rumor that you will soon be incapacitated.
- You do not want your prized stadium seats grabbed, or someone asking for your things, because *you won't be needing them anymore.*

When People Ask what they Can Do for You, Tell Them

Let people help you. It's a nice thing.

Accepting help is often part one of a two-part discussion. Have a list of things someone could do for you ready for the person to choose from. (The story about the Boy Scout who dragged a woman across a street she hadn't planned to cross comes to mind.)

There are those who ask if they can help out of courtesy, without expecting you to take them up on it. *Thanks* is all you need to say.

There are those whose help you don't want. *Thanks* is sufficient for them, too.

Consider Joining a Support Group

There are general cancer support groups and there are myeloma-specific groups. The value you get from attending support group meetings comes from an amazing and inventive collective wisdom. Patients and caregivers share discoveries and benefits. It is a special sort of insight you may not find anywhere else.

- Ask at your hospital. If it is one of those listed at the end of this chapter, all the contact names and phone numbers you need will be readily available. In fact, volunteers hoping to introduce new patients to support groups and to other free services will be roaming the patient waiting areas, looking for you.
- If you have joined the computing age, you will find myeloma support groups and blogs online. You can also access this treasure trove using a free computer—with free instruction if necessary—at your local public library.
- Or see *Meet Other Patients,* Chapter 4.

Get to Know One or More of the Nonprofits Standing by to Help You

The International Myeloma Foundation (IMF)

The IMF is the world's leading advocate in many areas of the fight against myeloma. It has a strong patient support arm. It tracks the locations and needs of myeloma support groups, providing information, pamphlets, and sometimes speakers. It can direct you to specialized resources, and it publishes free magazines in print and online. There's a hot line, 800-452-2873, providing answers to many patient questions, 9a.m. to 4p.m., Pacific Time, Monday through Friday.

The 800-phone number is an easy portal to everything the IMF offers if you do not have the ability to visit the nonprofit's excellent website, www.myeloma.org

There's no charge for anything.

The Multiple Myeloma Research Foundation (MMRF)

The MMRF was the first nonprofit to be primarily focused on helping myeloma patients. It raises more than $20 million a year, which it uses to encourage research. Together with its partners in the pharmaceutical industry and at academic centers, it has contributed to the development of six new treatments in the last decade and to the doubling of survival times for myeloma patients.

The MMRF also provides direct patient assistance.

For general patient information, go to www.themmrf.org. Also ask to receive *FastFacts,* a monthly e-newsletter and *MMRF Myeloma Focus,* a semi-annual newsletter. There are also events to learn about and to join.

To speak to a registered oncology nurse about the disease, treatments, supportive care, or clinical trials, call 866-603-6628 or go to patientnavigator@themmrf.org.

To find and contact a clinical trial, and then to enroll, visit www.myelomatrials.org.

Free, full-day educational symposia are offered for patients and caregivers at various places around the country. Go to www.themmrf.org/clinicalinsights to view the current schedule and to register.

The International Waldenstrom's Macroglobulinemia Foundation

The International Waldenstrom's Macroglobulinemia Foundation serves those with this much rarer form of bone cancer. The directors and officers of this organization are almost all patients, as well. Call 941-927-4963 or www.iwmf.com

Start a Clip File and a Library

In addition to your file with your prescriptions, test results, and receipts, you will find news articles about cancer in general and myeloma in particular. Some of them you will want to remember. There will be other books you will want to read and ear mark besides this one.

Treatment programs become complicated. They will be less difficult to manage if you start three-ring binders with all the information on each program in a place you can find later.

You may also want a binder with notes from the meetings of your support group. Include names and phone numbers of the friends you make there. Staple in the business cards of doctors and nurses who speak.

Everybody's a different sort of pack rat. The books you save and the articles that have value to you will change over time. Take nothing being suggested here as iron-clad. Just start the library and see where it goes. The only thing for sure is that you will find the trove of stuff you save valuable.

State	Location	Phone
AR	**Myeloma Institute for Research and Therapy** University of Arkansas, Little Rock myeloma.uams.edu	888-693-5662
AZ	**Samuel C. Johnson Medical Research Center** Mayo Clinic Cancer Center, Scottsdale www.mayoclinic.org/scottsdale	480-301-8000
CA	**Cancer Center and Beckman Research Institute** City of Hope, Duarte www.cityofhope.org	866-434-4673
CA	**Cedars-Sinai Medical Center** Los Angeles www.cedars-sinai.edu/Patients/Programs-and-Services/Multiple-Myeloma-and-Anyloidosis-Program	800-233-2771
CA	**Chao Family Comprehensive Cancer Center** University of California, Irvine www.cancer.uci.edu	714-456-3592

State	Location	Phone
CA	**Helen Diller Family Comprehensive Cancer Center** University of California, San Francisco cc.ucsf.edu	800-888-8664
CA	**Jonsson Comprehensive Cancer Center** University of California, Los Angeles www.cancer.ucla.edu	310-825-5268
CA	**Moores Cancer Center** University of California, San Diego cancer.ucsd.edu	858-534-7600
CA	**Stanford Cancer Center** Stanford University, Stanford cancer.stanford.edu/myeloma	650-498-6000
CA	**University of California Davis Cancer Center** University of California, Davis www.ucdmc.ucdavis.edu/cancer	800-362-5566
CA	**USC/Norris Comprehensive Cancer Center** University of Southern California, Los Angeles ccnt.hsc.usc.edu	800-872-2273
CO	**University of Colorado Cancer Center** Aurora www.uch.edu/conditions/cancer/blood-cancer-bmt/myeloma	800-473-2288
CT	**Yale Cancer Center** Yale University School of Medicine, New Haven yalecancercenter.org	203-688-4191

State	Location	Phone
DC	**Lombardi Comprehensive Cancer Center** Georgetown University Medical Center, Washington, DC lombardi.georgetown.edu	202-444-4400
FL	**H. Lee Moffitt Cancer Center & Research Institute** University of South Florida, Tampa moffitt.org	813-972-4673
FL	**Mayo Clinic Cancer Center** Jacksonville www.mayoclinic.org/multiple-myeloma	904-953-2272
GA	**Winship Cancer Institute** Emory University School of Medicine, Atlanta winshipcancer.emory.edu	888-9461447
IA	**Holden Comprehensive Cancer Center** University of Iowa, Iowa City www.uihealthcare.org	319-356-4200
IL	**Cancer Treatment Centers of America** Midwestern Regional Medical Center, Zion www.cancercenter.com/multiple-myeloma.cfm	800-931-0599
IL	**Robert H. Lurie Comprehensive Cancer Center** Northwestern University, Chicago cancer.northwestern.edu/home/index.cfm	866-587-4322
IL	**University of Chicago Comprehensive Cancer Center** Chicago cancer.uchicago.edu	888-824-0200

State	Location	Phone
IN	**Melvin & Bren Simon Cancer Center** Indianapolis cancer.iu.edu	888-600-4822
KS	**University of Kansas Hospital** Kansas City www.kumed.com	800-332-6048
MA	**Jerome Lipper Center for Multiple Myeloma** Dana-Farber Cancer Institute, Boston www.dana-farber.org/pat/adult/hematologic-oncology	617-632-3000
MD	**Johns Hopkins Oncology Center** Baltimore www.hopkinsmedicine.org/kimmel_cancer_center	410-502-1033
MD	**Marlene & Stewart Greenebaum Cancer Center** University of Maryland, Baltimore www.umgcc.org/hem_malig_program/canc_multmyel.htm	800-888-8823
MD	**National Cancer Institute, National Institute of Health** Bethesda www.cancer.gov/cancertopics/types/myeloma	800-422-6237
MI	**Barbara Ann Karmanos Cancer Institute** Wayne State University, Detroit www.karmanos.org	800-527-6266
MI	**University of Michigan Comprehensive Cancer Center** Ann Arbor mcancer.org	800-865-1125

State	Location	Phone
MN	**Masonic Cancer Center** University of Minnesota, Minneapolis www.cancer.umn.edu	612-624-8484
MN	**Mayo Clinic Cancer Center** Rochester www.mayoclinic.org/multiple-myeloma	507-284-2111
MO	**Siteman Cancer Center, Washington University Medical School** Barnes-Jewish Hospital, St. Louis www.siteman.wustl.edu	800-600-3606
NC	**Duke Comprehensive Cancer Center** Duke University Medical Center, Durham www.dukecancerinstitute.org	800-422-6237
NC	**Lineberger Comprehensive Cancer Center** The University of North Carolina, Chapel Hill unclineberger.org	866-828-0270
NC	**Wake Forest University Baptist Medical Center** Winston-Salem wakehealth.edu	800-446-2255
NE	**Eppley Cancer Center** University of Nebraska Medical Center, Omaha www.unmc.edu/cancercenter	402-559-4090
NH	**Norris Cotton Cancer Center** Dartmouth Hitchcock Medical Center, Lebanon www.cancer.dartmouth.edu	800-639-6918
NJ	**Cancer Institute of New Jersey** Robert Wood Johnson Medical School, New Brunswick cinj.org	732-235-2465

State	Location	Phone
NJ	**John Theurer Cancer Center** Hackensack University Medical Center, Hackensack www.jtcancercenter.org	201-996-5900
NY	**Albert Einstein Cancer Research Center** Albert Einstein College of Medicine, Bronx www.aecom.yu.edu/cancer	718-430-2302
NY	**Herbert Irving Comprehensive Cancer Center** NY Presbyterian Hospital/Columbia Presbyterian Center hiccc.columbia.edu	212-305-9327
NY	**Kaplan Comprehensive Cancer Center** NY University School of Medicine, New York cancer.med.nyu.edu	888-769-8633
NY	**Memorial Sloan-Kettering Cancer Center** New York www.mskcc.org	800-525-2225
NY	**Mount Sinai School of Medicine** New York www.mssm.edu	212-241-6500
NY	**Roswell Park Cancer Institute** Buffalo www.roswellpark.org	800-767-9355
NY	**St. Vincent's Comprehensive Cancer Center** Beth Israel Medical Center, New York www.myelomatreatment.org	888-4422623

State	Location	Phone
OH	**Cleveland Clinic** Cleveland my.clevelandclinic.org	800-223-2273
OH	**Ohio State University Myeloma Clinic** The James Cancer Hospital, Columbus cancer.osu.edu	614-293-7156
PA	**Abramson Cancer Center** University of Pennsylvania, Philadelphia www.penncancer.org	800-789-7366
PA	**Fox Chase Cancer Center** Philadelphia www.fccc.edu	215-728-2570
PA	**University of Pittsburgh Medical Center Cancer Center** Pittsburgh www.upci.upmc.edu	412-647-2811
TN	**Vanderbilt-Ingram Cancer Center** Vanderbilt University, Nashville www.vicc.org	615-936-1803
TX	**Charles A. Sammons Cancer Center at Dallas** Baylor University Medical Center, Dallas www.baylorhealth.com/SpecialtiesServices/transplantservices/pages/default.aspx	800-422-9567
TX	**M. D. Anderson Cancer Center** University of Texas, Houston www.mdanderson.org	800-392-1611
UT	**Huntsman Cancer Institute** University of Utah, Salt Lake City www.huntsmancancer.org	866-275-0243

State	Location	Phone
VA	**Cancer Center at the University of Virginia** Charlottesville www.healthsystem.virginia.edu/internet/cancer	800-223-9173
VA	**Virginia Cancer Specialists** Fairfax virginiacancerspecialists.com	703-208-3155
WA	**Fred Hutchinson Cancer Research Center** University of Washington, Seattle www.fhcrc.org	800-804-8824
WI	**Carbone Cancer Center** University of Wisconsin, Madison www.cancer.wisc.edu	608-262-5223
WI	**Medical College of Wisconsin** Milwaukee www.mcw.edu	414-955-3666

Notable Myeloma Treatment Centers

3

How to Be a Caregiver: Myeloma Is a Team Sport

Anita Chambers, Tammy Famularo, and Fern Tamkin

The government spends all kinds of time and money teaching test pilots how to be fearless. But they don't spend a goddamned penny teaching you how to be the fearless wife of a test pilot.

—Glennis Yeager (Barbara Hershey) to her famous test pilot husband, Chuck (Sam Shepard) in The Right Stuff

Greetings

We, who were drafted into this line of work ahead of you, now have 30 years of collective experience as caregivers to cancer patients, whom we also desperately love. We didn't train for this, nor would we ever want it. The hours can be very long. Conditions can be trying and stressful.

The Job Is Neither Complicated nor Heroic

We hope this is the first thing you have read about becoming a caregiver. We patient-groupies get taken awfully seriously by myeloma treatment teams. The result has been a proliferation of pompous psychosocial nursing pamphlets that are, frankly, embarrassing. Just use the KISS principle (Keep It Simple, Stupid)—and when all else fails, kiss the patient.

So Here You Are...

Welcome to test pilot flight school, featuring caregiver copilot training. All the thrills and challenges of pilot training and absolutely no control of anything.

You've got this person you love who's in trouble. Focus on how to be directly helpful. This will work best if you give the doctors and nurses your respectful close attention. Complement their great works. Make sure the patient follows their orders. But stay on the patient's side of the bed. The white coats are the healing team. You are patient support.

Listen to the doctors and nurses explain their quandaries. Be concerned, as they are, but trust them to come up with the best answers. Don't try to help them with your Internet discoveries or the advice of a friend.

Your job is to help the patient get to wherever the process sends the two of you. While there, you help the patient get through whatever it is that the professionals want to do to—or with—your patient. You listen to the doctor and you take notes. You see that prescriptions get filled and that other support chores get done. You go argue in the business office. You share the patient's worries. You may have to wipe the patient's chin. You do your best to keep the patient pain-free. Then you take the patient home, or back to the hospital room.

There will be times when you realize that one of the professionals treating your patient needs to know more about decisions or medications or history that took place somewhere else. Chime in. You're not the expert, but you think it may be important for the folks your patient is visiting to consult with another member of your patient's team. Have reports and phone numbers handy.

Be a Very Good Listener

Pay attention to your patient. Consciously focus and listen. If you have been married to the person for some time, be sure you are hearing what your spouse wants to say, not what you want to hear.

The person you're caring for is experiencing new ways that the human body can fail its inhabitant. Pain, disorientation, numbness, embarrassment, sight and hearing problems, other surprise malfunctions—and pride—are all taking a beating. You are the patient's first line of support. Pay your patient constant attention.

Don't presume that something you half heard is correct. Get the statement repeated. Check eyes and smiles for overall wellness messages.

The professionals ought to be better at careful communication but some are not. Learn how to get complete messages from each of those you are working with. If you have to, haul out a notepad or recorder.

Repeat back important instructions.

The Test Pilot Part of This

Everything that's good about myeloma treatment has been developed using trial and error—a process the medical community calls *clinical trial.* It is better than it sounds. Myeloma clinical trials over the past 40 years have brought us to a point where the disease has been, if not beaten, at least beaten back. Today, myeloma patients receiving proper care have futures.

You, as the caregiver, obviously want something with greater assurance for your guy or gal. The science just isn't there yet. Think of this as the fifth inning of a tied baseball game. We can win this thing but we haven't yet. Neither is it lost. Understand that the matter requires all the attention and resources possible. Stay on your toes. Clinical trials have brought us a long way and they bring us new victories all the time.

Helping Out: A Conversation with Fern Tamkin, Wife for 46 Years to Jim Tamkin, MD

"Of all the things I hear from friends, the least easy for me to deal with is, 'Please call me if there is anything I can do for you,'" says Fern. "These well-meaning gestures get really frustrating. They're adding tasks to a day that's already full. If I don't respond, that's slighting our friendship or keeping Jim's latest news a secret."

"Another thing," she continues, "how in heaven's name am I supposed to call the 30 friends who left messages on my answering machine while I was with Jim in the hospital? I know they mean well. They're really dears ... If I were the friend and they were the wife with the sick husband, it's probably what I would have done ... But just having to play through 30 messages, in case one of them is from one of Jim's doctors, is exasperating."

Fern shares two rules for being a helpful family member or friend:

1. Keep in touch but don't do it in ways that add to the caregiver's workload. Calling is fine but if you don't reach the person, weigh the possibility

that calling again may be easier on this person than leaving a message. If there's really no urgent need to talk, maybe send a card or flowers, or drop off something to eat.

2. Don't ask what you can do, suggest something. This makes it easier for the caregiver to respond.

Fern's cell phone rings in mid-sentence and she picks up. "Hello? Oh, yeah. Excuse me a minute, this is my sister. You're coming for dinner? Yes! Great idea! Stop by the market and get us some broccoli and maybe some salad greens."

She hangs up. The interlude has germinated a thought. "I have found that it helps our friends to give them things they can do for us. Run an errand. Buy the broccoli," she says.

Then she shares a rule for caregivers: "Don't try to do everything yourself. Friends and family want to help. Some need to help. Let them. Give those who love you the pleasure of being supportive. Relieve their frustrations by giving them something they can do."

"Later in this game, after you have become accustomed to your caregiver role, people will marvel and ask your advice," she offers finally. "Here's a good principle: each one teaches one. I've just taught you."

You Are Now the Expert

If you are a diligent caregiver, your patient's doctors will come to expect that you can answer their questions. Some of them are trivial: How about them Yankees? *No, we didn't watch the game. We go to bed about 9:30...*

Some of them matter a lot: Your patient's doctor tells you, *I don't understand this reaction. What meds is he taking now? Are you sure?*

> ...you are alone in the contestant's answer booth. A 30-second clock is counting down. You are wracking your brain to answer the $64,000 question, while a deranged stage manager pipes in deafening arpeggios from a 1950s Hammond Chord Organ...

Yeah, doc, I'm sure. Here is the current list of meds in our protocol, including OTC vitamins and pain killers.

Doctor-speak may not sound like you now, but it will. It comes naturally, by listening to what's going on and by keeping a few important records up to date.

Family Briefings

You and the patient also have a responsibility to keep friends and family apprised of events. Every caregiver–patient partnership develops its own style as to who goes first and says what. Often the caregiver talks most easily about the travails of the patient and the patient jokes about things the caregiver did or didn't do properly. However the duties of reporting are handed back and forth, family and friends need to hear from the two of you.

Please take these two terms, *need* and *responsibility,* to heart. They *need* to feel a part of the picture. You two are the only ones they can get good information from. So family briefings are a *responsibility.*

Reports by Post

Those who use the Internet will urge you and your patient to start some sort of website. It is a wonderful way to let people peek in to see how things are going without bothering you. But once started, you're on the hook to keep reports and maybe photos current.

The downside of using the Internet or social media, like Facebook, is that whatever one puts out *there* is open for both friends and the unscrupulous to use as they see fit. A possible solution to consider is at www.caringbridge.org. This is the service of a nonprofit foundation, offering free personal, protected sites where friends and family can share and receive support—a personalized caring social network—available 24/7. While everything is free, donations are gratefully accepted. More than a half a million people connect through Caring Bridge every day.

There Will Be Bad Days

There will be times when the patient hurts or hurts you. There will be days at the clinic when people screw up. There will be days when people shout at you or you shout at them. There will be days when you are terminally blue.

You have no idea what to do.

You need a buddy. The patient can't help.

If you are fortunate, there is a doc or nurse you have gotten close to at one of the places you and the patient visit. A phone call or a visit the next time you're there could be helpful.

Another place to get help is the support group you and the patient have joined. There may be a patient—more likely another patient's caregiver—that you as a fellow caregiver can talk to.

The hospital has a formal nursing program designed to be helpful. It also has volunteers and a team of psychiatrists who are there to help.

Take Care of Yourself

Substance abuse among family caregivers is relatively uncommon, experts report, but when it does occur, the stress of caregiving is almost always the root cause. At some point during the experience, at least a third of caregivers need counseling or some other sort of professional help to cope.

Stay at your best by taking breaks. Make a walk part of your daily routine. Prayer comes highly recommended. Spend time with a hobby or a job that has nothing to do with caregiving.

"One thing I would tell a new caregiver, watching someone go through this, is if you get depressed, go see someone about it," says Tammy Famularo, the veteran caregiver for her myeloma patient husband, Mark. "Which I finally did do after we had been going through this for several years ... I went to a support group for caregivers, sponsored by the Cancer Support Community. I also saw a therapist. Our church has also been a huge source of support and comfort."

While these resources have been helpful, Tammy had a further thought: "I would have been helped by having another caregiver who had been where I am, who I could phone to talk with. Even on a helpline. A nurse or a doctor would be less helpful. There were times in the middle of the night when I would just go down the hall and have a good cry."

See Tammy's List on p.38 for ways to connect with other patients and caregivers and read more of her and Mark's story in Chapter 15.

4

Meet Other Patients: Get to Know Your New Community

For survival's sake, find other patients and caregivers, and get to know them.

This Is a Practical Matter

If you have lived a mostly normal life till now, health needs have been the exception, not the rule. Your encounters with medical services carried with them the presumption that a condition would be addressed and settled. That has changed. Myeloma is here to stay.

You are the involuntary member of an exclusive club. You will benefit from finding other patients and caregivers who got here ahead of you. Meet, listen, share, benefit. Your dues will be cheaper.

Get a Patient's-Eye View of People and Places

Discuss your medical team with other patients. Get the best sense possible of who your key doctors and nurses are and how to work with them.

Some business offices have policies or procedures to learn about.

Find out about available facilities: the gym, pool, gift shop, cafeteria, ATM. In many hospitals, there is more than one place to eat. Quality, variety, and cost may be different.

Where's the cheapest parking? Can I get a handicapped parking permit? Is public transportation an option?

Concierge

Many hospitals now have concierge services. They're just like the guys in hotel lobbies. Ask them anything, they try to be helpful. No tip expected.

Drug Company Concierge

Several of the most important myeloma drug manufacturers offer free advice to myeloma patients through websites and toll-free hotlines. They include:

Celgene Patient Support Coordinator®	855-669-9630 www.celgene.com/patient-support/coordinator.aspx
Millennium Pharmaceuticals Velcade.com	866-835-2233 www.velcade.com
Novartis Patient Assistance Now	800-245-5356 www.patientassistancenow.com
Onyx Pharmaceuticals 360™	855-669-9630 www.onyx.com

Support Groups

Myeloma is a dangerous, complicated, difficult, scary, expensive thing. There are people—just like you—who have already *been there, done that,* and who will help you. Even if you are shy by nature, or very well known, or have some other reason for thinking you need anonymity, you can reduce the danger, simplify the situation, ease the difficulties, lessen the fear, and save on expenses by chatting about your experiences and needs in support group settings.

Ask your doctor or the hospital	There may be a name and phone number on your doctor's clipboard, or a pamphlet on a nearby literature rack. Most hospitals with myeloma treatment teams know where a nearby support group waits to help you.
International Myeloma Foundation	The IMF works with myeloma support groups throughout the nation. For one nearby, call 800-452-3873, or go to www.myeloma.org. Patient discussion helpline available.
The Leukemia and Lymphoma Society	800-955-4572 or www.lls.org. Chapters in major metropolitan areas across the nation. Each hosts patient and family support groups; some are myeloma-specific. Patient discussion helpline available.
Multiple Myeloma Research Foundation	Learn more about the disease, treatments, and clinical trials. 866-603-6628, or visit www.themmrf.org.
International Waldenstrom's Macroglobulinemia Foundation	941-927-4963 or www.iwmf.com. Experienced survivors answer the help line number and web address. Patient discussion helpline available.
Your church, temple, or mosque	Ask.
Cancer Support Community	888-793-9355 or www.cancersupportcommunity.org. Support groups across the country are sponsored. Patients with all sorts of cancer are served. Patient discussion helpline available.
The Internet	There are blogs by patients, organizational listings, and a multitude of other links and leads. This is the Wild West. The best and worst of information is side-by-side.

Patient and Family Seminars

The International Myeloma Foundation sponsors open meetings in a growing number of spots around the country each year. Distinguished panels of notables and professionals discuss advances in medical science and other matters of interest to myeloma patients. Call the IMF for a current schedule.

The Multiple Myeloma Research Foundation sponsors Clinical Insights, a series of free, full-day events for patients and caregivers. Call 866-603-6628, or visit www.themmrf.org/clinicalinsights to view the calendar and register.

Hospitals sometimes offer these events, too. Be careful not to confuse a meeting for patients with the continuing medical education (CME) programs that the docs and nurses go to. A meeting for patients will be low cost or free. The CME for professionals may come with a stiff tab. The CME will also be dense with technical jargon.

Regional myeloma groups also sponsor these get-togethers. The Arizona Myeloma Network, 623-388-6837, azmyelomanetwork.org, is notable. Also check with Multiple Myeloma Opportunities for Research & Education, 888-486-4240 or www.mmore.org.

Tammy's List

These contacts can match patients and caregivers for candid one-on-one sharing. All services are free.

The Anderson Network

M.D. Anderson Cancer Center's Network Patient and Caregiver Telephone Support Line can match you with a survivor with the same or a similar diagnosis, treatment, or experience, no matter where they received or are receiving treatment. Its aim—to connect those at different stages of the cancer journey so they can tap into each others' experiences—bridges the gap between patients who might not otherwise meet. It's also available to caregivers who'd like to speak with another caregiver of a patient similar to their own loved one. Telephone volunteers are screened and trained by Anderson Network staff and are encouraged to be a voice of hope and support, but not to give medical advice or to promote M.D. Anderson.

Call or use their online contact form.
Phone: 800-345-6324
www.mdanderson.org/patient-and-cancer-informat ion

4th Angel Mentoring Program

When diagnosed with testicular cancer in 1997, Olympic figure skating champion Scott Hamilton identified three "angels" who helped him. His oncology physician was his first angel, his oncology nurse was his second angel, and his family and friends were his third. What he found missing, however, was a fourth angel: someone who had gone through the same experience and who understood what he was feeling. Someone, in short, who had *been there.* After defeating his illness, Scott dedicated his life to promoting cancer research and awareness and to enlisting the help of a host of *angels* to support and comfort patients facing their own battle with cancer.

To that end, he launched the Scott Hamilton CARES Initiative and its first survivorship program—the 4th Angel Mentoring Program. Mentor matches are made based on age, gender, and diagnosis. Caregiver mentors are available as well and mentoring takes place via phone or e-mail.

Phone: 866-520-3197
www.4thangel.org

Imerman Angels

Jonny Imerman founded the organization in Chicago, remembering a day when he needed a quiet, candid conversation with someone who had been where he knew he was going, and who would give him some straight answers. When last we spoke with him, Imerman and his staff had recruited almost 5,000 cancer patients and caregivers around the world for his network. Call the number or visit the website; identify yourself and your need. Foundation staff will match you with a good person who will call you back.

Phone 866-IMERMAN
877-274-5529
312-274-5529
www.imermanangels.org

R.A. Bloch Cancer Foundation

The Bloch Cancer Foundation has more than 500 volunteer cancer survivors who offer support and information by sharing their perspectives. Cancer patients—or their supporters—can request a telephone call from someone who has survived the same diagnosis. Once you call or go online to fill out the "Match Me with a Survivor" form, you will be matched up as closely as possible with a volunteer survivor who will then call you.

Phone: 800-433-0464
www.blochcancer.org/contact/survivor-match

Blood & Marrow Transplant (BMT) Information Network

BMT's Caring Connections Program has more than 1,000 transplant survivors and family members who have volunteered to talk to others facing a transplant. In most cases, they can connect you with a survivor who had the same diagnosis, same type of transplant, and is approximately the same age as your patient.

Phone: 888-597-7674
www.bmtinfonet.org/services/support

CanCare

CanCare's mission is to improve the quality of life for cancer patients and their families by providing one-on-one, long-term emotional and spiritual support from trained volunteers who have experienced and survived the same cancer diagnosis or who have been caregivers to someone who has. Generally, support is provided over the phone and sometimes through e-mail, and those who are matched with someone in the same geographical area are encouraged to make an effort to meet in person.

Phone: 888-461-0028
www.cancare.org/look-for-support.asp

Cancer Hope Network

Cancer Hope Network provides free and confidential one-on-one support to cancer patients and their families by matching them with trained volunteers who have themselves undergone and recovered from a similar cancer experience. If you would like to be matched with a Support Volunteer, call or submit your match request online. Their staff will initiate a search, discuss the results of the search with you, and make a recommendation as to the Support Volunteer who most closely mirrors your situation. The Support Volunteer will call you within 48 hours.

Phone: 800-552-4366

www.cancerhopenetwork.org/index.php?page=find amatch

Leukemia and Lymphoma Society

The Patti Robinson Kaufmann First Connection Program is a peer-to-peer program that links newly diagnosed patients and their families with trained volunteers who have been touched firsthand by a blood cancer and who have shared similar experiences. You must first call or go online to get your local Leukemia and Lymphoma Society chapter's patient services manager, who will then match you with a trained peer volunteer based on diagnosis, age, and gender when possible. Your peer volunteer will then arrange for one or two phone calls or meetings with you at a mutually convenient time and place. The information shared between a trained peer volunteer and a patient or family member is strictly confidential.

Phone: 800-955-4572
www.lls.org/FirstConnection

5

The Cognoscenti: Your Treatment Team

You are the reason for a tribal gathering.

The Selection Circumstance

You didn't really choose your *cognoscenti*—your medical team—any more than somebody in a car wreck chose which paramedics showed up. A physician or a nurse recognized your need for an oncologist and sent you to one. And so the gathering began.

Others came along as circumstances prescribed, as when your oncologist said, "I'm sending you to Radiation for an evaluation..." which is how you acquired your radiation oncologist. Then someone said, "Get this prescription filled and I'll see you in a week...." Voila! A drug manufacturer who will play an important role in your recovery just joined your team, along with a pharmacist.

This fortuitous team-building is reasonable under the circumstances. The people stepping out of the woodwork to help you know this game and you don't. You're on autopilot, which is very fortunate since you have none of the necessary skills to fly this plane. Nevertheless, it is your flight. You should know who these people are and you should feel at home with them.

The Cognoscenti

Cognoscenti began the practice of organizing themselves into professional circles in ancient China, Greece, and Rome. The cognoscenti we care about chose medicine. Others focused on banking, music, art, food,[2] or crime.[3] Each has a common, consuming herd interest. You entered the world of the healing tribe when you became sick. You will live there at least part time for the foreseeable future.

Here, in alphabetical order, are cognoscenti that myeloma patients encounter.

Acupuncturist

Acupuncture is a therapeutic technique that originated in China 5,000 years ago. It encourages the body to promote natural healing, or to improve functioning. This is done by manipulating thin, solid needles that have been inserted into very precise points in the

---

2 The foodies adopted their own name, connoisseur, from cognoscenti.

3 The Godfather has roots.

skin, sometimes accompanied by heat or electrical stimulation.

Acupuncture is used in pain control and relief from neuropathy for myeloma patients.

A person offering this skill must have a master's degree in acupuncture or in oriental medicine. These academic programs, including internship, generally take three to four years to complete.

There is a related art, *acupressure,* which practices the same skills without penetrating the skin. Physical therapists, chiropractors, and osteopaths also use it.

Chiropractor

Chiropractic health care is concerned with the diagnosis, treatment, and prevention of disorders of the *neuromusculoske letal* system and the effects of these disorders on general health. Think interactions between nerves, muscles, and bones.

Chiropractors are also trained to recommend therapeutic and rehabilitative exercises, as well as to provide nutritional, dietary, and lifestyle counseling.

> Since bone disease is the common complaint of all myeloma patients, chiropractic care can be a controversial decision, though as a patient, I have found it gives me great relief.
>
> *—Jim Tamkin, MD*

Following attainment of an undergraduate degree, chiropractic college lasts three to four years. The World Health Organization has stated that no less than 4,200 hours of schooling in a chiropractic college is required to become a doctor of chiropractic.

Dentist

Dentists study, diagnose, prevent, and treat diseases, disorders, and conditions of the mouth, the jaw, adjacent associated organs and structures, and their impact on the rest of you.

Drugs used in myeloma treatments may cause damage in areas your dentist needs to help you with. The mouth is also a prime point of entry for germs. Your dentist needs to know what's going on during periods when your immune system has been compromised by myeloma or its drug treatments. Very nasty infections can start in the mouth. Your jawbone can be compromised. *Osteonecrosis,* bone death, is a threat to myeloma patients during chemo. Teeth may be attacked. Sores or even boils may appear in the mouth and on the tongue.

Dentists complete undergraduate and doctoral degree programs in about eight years. A few dentists go on to add oral surgery or oncology to their areas of expertise. Extra degrees requiring as much as a decade of further work may be necessary.

Hematologist

Hematology is the study of blood, blood-forming organs, and blood diseases. A *hematologist* is a physician who specializes in the diagnosis, treatment, and prevention of blood and bone marrow diseases, and who also studies immunologic, hemostatic (blood clotting), and anemia disorders.

Myeloma is a blood disease. Many oncologists who treat it have hematology as a second specialty.

Hematologists are required to complete a four-year bachelor's degree, a four-year medical school degree and between two and four years of postgraduate clinical fellowship.

Herbalist

Herbal medicine uses plants to treat or prevent disease and promote health. It is practiced by a range of health professionals, including chiropractors and naturopathic doctors. Although there are dedicated herbal medicine schools to train would-be herbalists, the practice of using plants as remedies is traditional in many cultures, each of which has its own criteria for training and certification.

Herbalists must learn many skills, including the cultivation of herbs, the diagnosis and treatment of conditions, and the dispensing and preparation of herbal medications.

To become a practicing herbalist, the American Herbalists Guild recommends a program of at least 1,600 hours of study at a school of herbal medicine, including 400 hours in a clinic.

Naturopathic physicians must complete a bachelor's degree as well as a four-year Doctor of Naturopathic Medicine program.

Infectious Diseases Physician

From time to time, all myeloma patients need physicians who specialize in infection fighting. Side effects of chemotherapy are particularly notorious for weakening the immune system. Infection marches in. You'd be in *deep serious* without your ID doc.

Native American Healer

Native American medicine is a broad term that includes the healing beliefs and practices of hundreds of indigenous North American tribes. This form of healing combines religion, spirituality, herbal medicine, and rituals that are used to treat people with medical and emotional conditions. From the Native American perspective, medicine is more about healing the whole person than about curing a specific disease. Traditional healers aim to *make whole* by restoring well-being and harmonious relationships with the community and the spirit of nature.

Native American healing has been around for centuries. Many of its practices were outlawed and then restored to legitimacy in 1978 on the grounds that restriction violated freedom of religion.

Nephrologist

Nephrologists are physicians specializing in kidney diseases, transplants, and dialysis. Their primary goal is to diagnose medical problems of the kidneys and find ways to maintain or restore kidney function. Other than performing biopsies of kidneys, a nephrologist does not perform surgery, referring surgical candidates to urologists.

Most myeloma patients suffer kidney disease as the result of either the cancer or the drugs used to combat it. One in five myeloma patients will experience kidney failure.

Most nephrologists complete eight years of college and graduate education, a three-year residency in internal medicine, and another two years of training specifically in kidney-related conditions. A specialty within the field of nephrology, such as oncology, requires additional training and certification.

Nurse

Nursing focuses on the care of individuals, families, and groups so that they may attain, maintain, or recover optimal health and quality of life. The first level of professional attainment is to become a licensed practical nurse (LPN) or licensed vocational nurse (LVN). A registered nurse (RN) has graduated from a nursing program at a college or university and has passed a national licensing exam. An elite group obtain a PhD in a field of special interest within nursing. Others become nurse practitioners, with many of the responsibilities and privileges of physicians, including authority to prescribe most drugs.

Generally, an LPN or LVN degree can be earned in a year. An RN designation can be earned with an associate degree in nursing, which takes two years. A bachelor of science in nursing (BSN) takes four years. A master's degree in nursing requires at least one year of study after obtaining a BSN. Most states also require continuing education to keep a nursing license current.

An oncology certified nurse designation, is reserved for a RN who has served for at least a year as an RN has completed specialized coursework, has done 1,000 hours of cancer patient care, and has passed an examination administered by the Oncology Nursing Certification Corporation. Oncology nurses may administer radiation therapy, antibiotics, chemotherapy, and blood transfusions to patients.

Be very good to your nurses. They run the show.

Nutritionist

Weight loss, particularly unexplained weight loss, will concern your doctor. It is presumed to be the result of either myeloma's aggressive behavior or a side effect of one of the drugs you are taking. Blood tests will reveal any specific area of malnutrition that should be rectified. A nutritionist will work with you on menus, the number of meals to eat each day, and related matters.

The most recognized credential for a nutritionist is registered dietitian, which is accredited by the American Dietetic Association's Commission on Accreditation for Dietetics Education.

> Do differences in diet account for the fact that black Americans get myeloma twice as often as white Americans? no. Nor do the culinary proclivities of Asians explain why they get myeloma less often than Caucasians.

Oncologist

Your lead physician, your oncologist, has earned several college degrees, served a four-to eight-year internship, and probably went on to specialize in the study of your illness, a branch of a subspecialty that is insanely complicated.

Oncology is derived from the ancient Greek, *onkos*—meaning bulk, mass, or tumor. Add the suffix, *logy*—meaning study of. It is the branch of medicine that deals with cancer.

So you come home from seeing this person and your daughter says to you, "How'd you like Dr. Doe?"

And you say, "She's good. I like her."

Translation: Your daughter said to you, *Is this person someone you can be comfortable with? Do you plan to trust this person with your life?*

And you replied, *I guess so, Honey.*

Ophthalmologist

An *ophthalmologist* is a specialist in medical and surgical problems dealing with the anatomy, physiology, and diseases of the eye.

Ophthalmologists are medical doctors who have completed a college degree, medical school, and four years of residency training, with the first year being an internship in surgery, internal medicine, pediatrics, or a general transition year. Optional fellowships in advanced topics may be pursued for several years after residency.

You should visit an ophthalmologist before and after chemotherapy due to the possibility that your drugs may cause cataracts or other eye problems. You want to preserve your eye health, of course. You also want to establish the condition of your eyes before you began the treatment so that your insurance company will have positive proof of cause if you must file a claim for collateral damage from chemo drugs.

Osteopath

Two co-equal sorts of physicians practice medicine in the United States. Most hold the Doctor of Medicine degree (MD). Osteopathic physicians hold the Doctor of Osteopathic Medicine degree (DO). The medical training for an MD and DO is pretty much the same, though osteopathic manipulative medicine (OMM), a type of manual therapy taught only at DO schools, sets them apart.

OMM takes into account the physical and mental health of a patient and how either aspect, or both aspects, could be contributing to the disease state. A DO is trained to perform a structural diagnosis and integrate it into the entire history and physical exam process and to use osteopathic manipulative technique (OMT) when appropriate. Using OMT, an osteopathic physician will move your muscles and joints with stretching, gentle pressure, and resistance.

While osteopathy emphasizes the role of the musculoskeletal system and focuses on preventive health care, it also incorporates drugs and surgery.

Both MDs and DOs complete four-year postgraduate programs, and must pass the same licensing exam to be admitted to practice. DO physicians complete conventional residencies in hospitals and training programs, are licensed in all states, and have rights and responsibilities identical to those of MDs.

Pharmacist

Pharmacists are responsible for providing us with safe and effective drugs. Compounding pharmacists have a special license permitting them to mix custom medications to a physician's specifications.

Your druggist serves you from behind the scenes during chemotherapy, radiation, and at other points in your journey. The safety and effectiveness of clinical trials are often dependent on the skills and knowledge of the pharmacist.

Pharmacists are paying attention to your overall treatment program and looking for possible unintended drug interactions, consequences of the IVs, and handfuls of drugs, vitamins, and herbs you take.

In the United States, a Doctor of Pharmacy degree requires completion of four years at an accredited college of pharmacy after obtaining an undergraduate bachelor's degree. Pharmacists are educated in pharmacology, chemistry, organic chemistry, biochemistry, pharmaceutical chemistry, microbiology, pharmaceutics, pharmacy law, physiology, anatomy, pharmacokinetics, pharmacodynamics, drug delivery, pharmaceutical care, and compounding of medications.

Additional curriculum areas may cover diagnosis with emphasis on laboratory tests, disease state management, therapeutics, and the process of selecting the most appropriate medication for a given patient.

Phlebotomist

A nurse or technician may use this title, which refers to a person with special training in the taking of blood samples and blood-related fluids, including bone marrow. Two hundred years ago, phlebotomists were physicians who believed that they could relieve disease and fever by opening a vein, allowing blood to carry the malady out of the patient's body. As we know today, the theory was flawed. Our country's first president, George Washington, was bled to death by phlebotomists.

Physical Therapist

Physical therapy, also called *physiotherapy,* is used to fix impairments and disability. It also promotes healing and mobility. In many settings, physical therapy services are provided alongside, or in conjunction with, other medical or rehabilitation services.

Definitions and licensing requirements vary among jurisdictions. Each state has enacted its own physical therapy practice act. The American Physical Therapy Association (APTA) has drafted a national standard for its members.

The APTA is responsible for accrediting physical therapy education. A two-year associate degree for physical therapist assistants is the minimum requirement for those in this profession whom you will encounter in hospitals. Many physical therapists hold nursing and other degrees.

Psychiatrist

A physician practicing psychiatry specializes in the diagnostic evaluation and psychopharmacological treatment of mental disorders. Only psychiatrists are authorized to prescribe psychiatric medication, conduct psychiatric examinations, and order and interpret laboratory tests for psychiatric patients.

In the United States, one must complete a bachelor's degree and four years of medical school to earn an MD or DO. The candidate must then practice as a psychiatric resident for four years. This training includes comprehensive diagnosis, psychopharmacology, medical care issues, and psychotherapies.

Radiologist

Radiology is a physician's specialty that uses imaging to diagnose and treat the body. Radiologists use an array of imaging technologies, including x-rays, ultrasound, computed tomography, nuclear medicine, positron emission tomography, and magnetic resonance imaging.

A radiologist may use imaging to guide the instruments of surgeons more accurately. This permits whole new levels of minimally invasive work. You benefit because surgery is safer and you recover more quickly. As examples, vascular and organ procedures that until very recently required months of recovery can now require only days for recovery, because the doctors use image-guided arms to reach the area of repair through arteries instead of opening the chest.

Radiologists must complete undergraduate education, four years of medical school, one year of internship, and four years of residency training. After residency, radiologists often pursue one or two years of additional specialty fellowship training.

Radiation Oncologist

A *radiation oncologist* is a doctor who specializes in the treatment of cancer patients, using radiation therapy as the main modality of treatment. Radiation can be used to destroy cancer, either alone or in combination with surgery and chemotherapy. It may also be used to reduce pain.

The course work for a radiation oncologist is the same as for a radiologist, but more oncology training is added.

Surgeon

All myeloma patients experience surgery. It is mostly minor, outpatient stuff, but major procedures can be called for. Co-morbidities—additional disorders or conditions you may have, such as cataracts—may also demand surgery. For more information, see Chapter 14, *Notes on Surgery: Surgery Plays Supporting Roles.*

Urologist

Urologists apply general and surgical skills to relieve symptoms and to correct abnormalities of the urinary tract, bladder, and kidneys. They also specialize in therapies for male reproductive organs.

Urologists must finish a bachelor's degree, medical school, and five years of residency before becoming board certified.

Getting Down to Business

As the circumstances of your health problem become clearer, the cognoscenti become more numerous. If someone in the group is not right for you, or if you see that one person clashes with others, you have a responsibility to see that things are either smoothed over or that a replacement is found.

Are we telling you that you may have to pick and choose among highly exalted professionals? Even though you have no way to evaluate their skills? Yes.

You will probably discuss the matter with another of the cognoscenti that you have come to trust, then be guided by a mutual decision. But, yes, you should step up to this. You must have a compatible team: a group that works tirelessly, seamlessly, cooperatively, selflessly, on your behalf.

That Gut Feeling

Trust your instinct and common sense. A person who lets you cool your heels in his or her office for an hour or two every time you visit, and never shows the slightest embarrassment, may be telling you something important about the value placed on you and on your well-being.

A person who refuses to consult with others on your team may be indicating a lack of trust, which could affect cohesion. Politics and code of tribal conduct may keep one doctor from talking to another about it. That leaves you to bring the team conflict up and broker a settlement.

If you ever get the impression that somebody thinks they have you trapped—that you have no choice but to be treated in one office, or by one individual—ask a pointed question. If your impression is confirmed, bail. These people are promising to neglect you.

A person who is cold and distant, especially when it causes him or her to have trouble communicating with you, is missing an attribute that you sorely need.

Maybe you can work with this person. Maybe you can't. Trust your gut.

Part Two

Financial and Workplace Issues

6

Health Insurance and Other Benefits: Your Financial Safety Net

Know your options and plan for obstacles.

Health Insurance

Qualifications

The sort of financial shelter available to you pivots on four variables: your age, your employment status, a Social Security number, and any health insurance you had before you got sick.

- If you have health insurance, you've got your ticket. Your coverage has recently been improved by federal government fiat. Exclusions and caps should have been eliminated, though you must check to be sure.
- If you are age 65 or above and you have a Social Security number, you've got Medicare. You're good to go.
- If you work full time for an employer with more than 50 workers, you're covered. You have either a health maintenance organization (HMO) or a preferred provider organization (PPO). "There are only two key things to know: the costs that co-pays and deductibles leave for you to cover and where the boundaries of your service network are," advises Dean R. Zimmerman, Zimmerman Financial & Insurance Services in Torrance, California. HMOs and PPOs feature networks of doctors and treatment centers. You are expected to choose from among the resources in your plan—and only those resources—when seeking medical care. And no others.

  The complexities of treating myeloma almost guarantee that the time will come when something or someone beyond the boundaries of your HMO or PPO is needed for you. Yor insurance provider can make provision for it. Leave the normal bounds of your plan *only* as instructed by your insurance provider so that you retain all of your provider's benefits.

- If you are younger than 65, have a Social Security number, no insurance but enough money to buy a policy, call your state insurance commissioner or the American Cancer Society, 800-227-2345. Find out how the uninsured buy coverage in your state; it will be either a state-run health insurance exchange or something similar. Look over the plans and options. Buy one. Starting January 1, 2014, you could no longer be denied insurance due to a pre-existing condition. There may, however, be a waiting period until your policy is in full, unconditional force.
- If you are younger than 65, have a Social Security number, and your income is limited, you may be eligible for Medicaid (visit www.Medicaid.gov) or subsidized private insurance (apply for a subsidy when you buy your insurance). Medicaid involves many rules and requirements, but it is coverage.

No Social Security Number

If you don't have a Social Security number, contact one of the law firms that specialize in this predicament. Many of them are listed online and in the Yellow Pages as immigration law specialists. Of the several ways to get the number, and thereby to qualify for health insurance, legal counsel is fastest and most user friendly. There is a fee. It may be negotiable.

Free legal resource teams are a distant second best. They take too much time—months—to help you. If you have any special circumstances, you may find that you are handed back to a fee-based legal service anyway.

Cancer Legal Resource Center	866/843-2572
Patient Advocate Foundation	800/532-5274

Some other avenues:

- Your congressional district office may have specialists who understand your predicament and are able to help you.
- Your city and county offices may also have resources for you.
- Most law schools offer pro bono help that you can get by calling the school's main phone number.
- Many community advocate groups also provide lawyers to help with this issue.

How to Get Your Health Insurance Started

You started the insurance process when you and a doctor discovered your disease. That clipboard of forms the receptionist handed you included the health insurer's necessary paperwork. You're launched.

If your insurance situation is uncertain, you're still launched. A procedure has begun that the appropriate insurance people and your health care team will help you with. Be trusting. Everybody wants to support you. When the paperwork becomes exasperating, relax, take a deep breath, and then go back at it. Being accurate and thorough is serious business. A mountain of money is on the table. If it is any consolation, your end of the paperwork pales by comparison to your medical team's stack.

Don't Stir Up the Health Care Insurance Administrators

Your health insurance policy may have come with a pamphlet that gives you instructions about first things to do to start treatment coverage. Or some friend, hearing about your diagnosis, may have a strongly-held opinion as to who you need to contact—*right away!*

"Don't do it," advises Zimmerman. Start the health care insurance coverage process by going to your doctor for treatment, just as described in the preceding segment. Let your doctor's people take it from there. They're better at it than you would be. They're faster. They know what to say and who to say it to.

Insurance and Newly Developed Treatments

Some of the best minds in medicine are helping you fight your disease. New things are constantly being considered. Some of them are too new for your insurance people to automatically agree to pay for. Whenever a new drug is introduced to you, or a new procedure is contemplated, ask if it is acceptable to your health insurance team. If it isn't, any of several warning flags are being raised. Cost is only one of them. Make sure you are completely comfortable with this treatment and its side effects, as well as who pays for what.

How to Fix Medicare and Medicaid Disputes

In California, Della Saavedra, a myeloma Medicaid patient, was summarily plucked from her successful City of Hope treatment program and reassigned to L.A. Care. This was part of a mandate from Obamacare to get two million of the nation's sickest into cheaper treatment.

"L.A. Care had no idea what to do with me," she says. By chance, she found a legal aid firm that took her case. After a year of letters, tears, and litigation, she's back in competent hands at City of Hope.

If you are served by Medicare or Medicaid and this happens to you:

Medicare Appeals

MAXIMUS Federal Services

585-425-5200

Medicaid Appeals

MAXIMUS State Appeals Project

866-763-6395

Other Benefits

Disability

If sickness is putting you out of work, you may be eligible for either state or federal disability insurance benefits. Several states provide disability programs that are funded by mandatory employee contributions; California, Hawaii, New Jersey, New York, and Rhode Island. If you live in one of the other states, you'll be working with either a group or private disability insurance provider. Your doctor's staff will be your best advisor as to what should be done next, and how to contact the folks who do this for you.

You could also be eligible to receive Social Security Disability Income (SSDI) from the United States Social Security Administration. This is provided for those who have worked in the past, but have since become unable to work due to a disability. You must have contributed to Social Security at some point in your life in order to be eligible, and the benefit amount is dependent on your earnings record with Social Security. If disability puts you out of work, you may get up to 60% of your base pay, tax-free, until Social Security kicks in.

If you qualify for disability status, you may be able to get health insurance faster, cheaper, and regardless of your age, through Medicare, with little or no pre-existing disease waiting period. Because Social Security and Medicare eligibility rules are complex, you should call Social Security at 800-772-1213 to get the most accurate information regarding your particular situation.

You also get one of those nifty handicapped parking passes, free parking in metered areas in some cities, and toll-free passage on roads and bridges, among other goodies.

Veterans and surviving spouses may be able to get the help they need more quickly or more cheaply from the Department of Veterans Affairs (VA).

You may also qualify for a military disability pension. You must be a wartime veteran with limited income and you must be unable to work or be age 65 or older.

Help from the VA will not disqualify you from getting SSDI, nor will it affect the amount you can receive. Each program is wholly separate. Get the max from both.

The Agent Orange (and Other Herbicides) Special Circumstance—For Both Military and Civilians in the Department of Defense

Those who served in places where herbicides were used for broad area defoliation may qualify for VA disability compensation, medical care, and other benefits. The VA presumes that your myeloma was caused by the chemicals. You do not have to provide evidence of exposure, or even to have known that these leaf killers were being used.

Qualifying Areas of Service

- Vietnam at any time, no matter how brief, during the war (1962–1975).
- If you served in the Navy offshore from Vietnam, in any of the Coast Guard's Southeast Asia missions, or you served in Thailand (1962–1975), you should apply.
- Those stationed near the Korean Demilitarized Zone between April 1968 and August 1971 are eligible.

- If you were stationed at Fort Detrick or Fort Drum, New York, in 1959.
- Everybody else who served anywhere that stored Agent Orange or trained with it.

Downwinders

If you were around in the 1950s, you may remember the innocence of the era. Bleachers were set up for the comfort of those gathered to watch atomic bombs go off. Heavily smoked glass was passed out, encouraging people to stare directly at the explosion. Observation sites were located just far enough away to keep people from being hurt by flying debris and blast wave heat.

Gambling sometimes stopped in Las Vegas so that everyone could go outside to watch the horizon light up. Elsewhere in America's great southwestern desert, folks went on about their normal lives, generally unconcerned by the occasional flash and rumble.

Buck Sergeant Jesse DeLeon was one of a company of Marines dug in about three miles from a Desert Rock, Nevada, test site in 1954. The flash was so bright he could see the outline of bone through the flesh in his hand. Just after the blast wave passed over the top of his trench, DeLeon's unit formed up and marched through ground zero. "There was a weird, warm feeling," he remembers.

Every few years, Jesse gets a note from the Pentagon wondering how he's doing health wise. Other than the bother of arthritis, the 75-year-old owner of Jesse DeLeon's Hair Design in Torrance, California, is just fine. He is also acutely aware of how lucky he is.

The Radiation Exposure Compensation Act (RECA)

Aboveground nuclear weapons tests in southern Nevada, beginning in the 1940s, caused everyone living in the region ("downwinders") to be exposed to radiation. Parts of Arizona and Utah were also lit up. Congress adopted the RECA in October 1990, to help those who were poisoned.

Document your condition for the Department of Justice's Civil Division, Torts Branch, to get a tax-free settlement check:[4]

---

4 According to RECA, a myeloma patient—even one who has succumbed—who lived in any of the following counties for a period of at least two years between January 21, 1951, and October 31, 1958, or during the entire month of July 1962, may qualify for tax-free compensation: In Arizona—Apache, Coconino, Gila, Navajo, Yavapai. In Nevada—Eureka, Lander, Lincoln, Nye, White Pine, or the northern portion of Clark. In Utah—Beaver, Garfield, Iron, Kane, Millard, Piute, San Juan, Sevier, Washington, or Wayne.

- $50,000 to individuals residing or working downwind of the Nevada test site
- $75,000 for workers participating in above ground nuclear weapons tests

Atomic Veterans

If you participated in a *radiation-risk activity* while in uniform, you are what the VA unofficially calls an atomic veteran:

- Participated in the occupation of Hiroshima and Nagasaki, Japan, between August 6, 1945, and July 1, 1946
- Was a prisoner of war in Japan during World War II
- Served in the vicinity of atmospheric nuclear weapons tests in Nevada and the Pacific Ocean between 1945 and 1962

You are also atomic if you participated in underground nuclear weapons testing on Amchitka Island, Alaska, before January 1, 1974.

You are atomic if you worked for at least 250 days before February 1, 1992, at a gaseous diffusion plant in Paducah, Kentucky; in Portsmouth, Ohio; or at K25 in Oak Ridge, Tennessee.

You don't have to prove a connection between myeloma and the place you served; only that you have myeloma and that you were at one of those places. Surviving spouses, dependent children, and dependent parents of atomic veterans may be eligible for survivors' benefits:

- Tax-free disability compensation of $2,500 per month, in addition to Social Security disability benefits
- Free medical, dental, and vision care at any VA treatment center
- Free drugs
- Free medical coverage for your spouse and dependents through CHAMPVA, the retired military family plan
- Free access to military BX, PX, and commissaries
- Waiver of vehicle licensing fee in most states
- Reduction or elimination of property tax obligations
- Access to military recreation and lodging facilities at reduced rates
- Educational benefits for yourself and your dependents
- A $10,000 term life insurance policy
- Free burial in a military cemetery and free headstone
- Waiver of the 2% fee for a VA home loan

- Disabled parking privileges in most places

Overseas Treatment Options

Some countries and some foreign hospitals will bid competitively to get you to leave America for treatment. They do this because your health insurance benefits are transferable, and because the rates that can be charged to Medicare or your private carrier are lucrative. They also profit by the dollar exchange on U.S. Government and private corporate retirement benefits.

Detractors may point out that the quality of care elsewhere is lower than you would receive in the United States. Check it out. The claim may—or may not be—true.

Investigate "Medical Tourism"

There is a growing movement by large employers, fed up with wildly varying price tags, to offer generous incentives to fly ailing employees to an excellent hospital for a cut-rate group deal on a very expensive procedure, such as a transplant. In 2012, grocery giant Kroger flew nearly two dozen workers to a Southern California medical center for orthopedic work. Wal-Mart Stores, Inc., began offering employees and their dependents travel deals in 2013. Ask your employer's health care administrator or your insurance carrier if there are any specials you should know about.

On the international scene, Hadassah University Medical Center, Jerusalem, Israel, is now expanding to treat a broader clientele from across the Mediterranean and throughout the Middle East. It welcomes American patients, offering remarkable, state-of-the-art oncology with lower out-of-pocket costs to visitors from the United States. A concierge service is under consideration that would bundle in luxury hotel accommodations and tours of historical points of interest. Get your transplant for much less *and* visit the Wall of the Temple Mount. The service may even send a private jet for new patients at some point in the future.

Switzerland, Thailand, Mexico, Singapore, Panama, Grenada, Belize, other Caribbean nations, and the Cook Islands, among a growing list of others, may also offer oncology in exotic settings. Look for them to do deals with your health insurance provider.

> Foreign government-run health care systems that are highly socialized—including several that aggressively promote free health care to both U.S. English and Spanish speakers—have waiting periods before treatment and maximum age limits on some procedures that myeloma patients count on. Let's not be subtle here. You could get there and find out that you are too old to qualify for the procedure or drugs you need, or that you must wait a length of time for treatment that is tantamount to a death sentence.

Nobody Throws Money Around Like a Myeloma Patient

The sums of money required for treatment of myeloma are obscene: $100 pills. $2,500 shots. $50,000 chemo. $80,000 kidney dialysis. $100,000 *minor* surgeries. Quarter of a million for a stem cell transplant. You are obviously not going to take care of what you will need out of the egg money.

Under the best of circumstances, you can expect to lay out $6,000 for annual out-of-pocket spending and more for your share of insurance premiums and co-pays. You will also write checks for things that are not covered by health insurance. There are likely to be attractive services offered by people and organizations that do not participate in insurance and federal healthcare umbrella programs. Some of these costs can be deducted from income at tax time (see Chapter 8, Myeloma Tax Savings: Minimize Your Tax Burden and Get Some Money Back).

For more help with costs, go on to Chapter 7, Low-Hanging Fruit.

7

Low-Hanging Fruit: Financial Help, Free Services, and Discount Drugs

Drug companies offer discounts and nonprofits have stipends as high as $10,000 that you can apply for.

There are discounts to help with your astronomically priced pharmaceuticals. There are other funds that help with the fees and the unpaid portions of the innumerable other expenses related to dealing with this disease. This chapter's tips and tactics should make life a little easier on your wallet.

Tip #1—Don't keep financial hardship a secret.

When you're talking to someone and they ask you a question about how you are doing or what's going on, explain to them what's going on. I was diagnosed in August, which meant that with my insurance, between August and the end of the year I was going to have to pay a $10,000 deductible and $5,000 out of pocket. When I was talking with my best friend, he asked what was going on, so I told him. We didn't talk any more about it, but *about a week before Christmas he called me and said, "I'm going to send you something FedEx. Are you going to be home?" I said "Yeah." The next day I got a check for over $15,000 via FedEx. He had canvassed my graduating high school class—there were only 120 of us—and they had taken up more than $15,000 to cover my deductible and out-of-pocket. So when people ask, tell 'em. Tell 'em what's going on.*

—Carl

Multiple myeloma patient

Wellness Community testimony

Redondo Beach, CA

It is *very* unwise to hope for help from friends or family. Nevertheless, based on the volume of reports like Carl's, it seems short-sighted to keep financial needs a secret.

Tip #2—There are organizations that are in the business of helping you with co-pays and other incidental expenses.

These programs help pay for the out-of-pocket expenses you are left with after insurance pays most of the bill. Some of the programs also assist with insurance premiums and co-pay deductibles.

Contacting the individual programs will give more information to determine what is covered as well as eligibility requirements. If you have any doubt as to how to ask for help, amounts that are realistic, necessary proofs of cost or of eligibility, follow these programs' guidelines carefully. If you need more help, phone the organization and ask someone before submitting your request.

Chronic Disease Fund, Inc.

Chronic Disease Fund, Inc., helps those who cannot afford the medications prescribed for them. It specifically defrays unpaid portions of Kyprolis, Pomalyst, Revlimid, Thalomid, and Velcade up to a figure that varies from year to year. In 2013, the ceiling was $7,000.

www.cdfund.org
6900 N. Dallas Parkway, Suite 200
Plano, TX 75024
Phone: 877-YOUR-CDF (968-7233)

HealthWell Foundation

The HealthWell Foundation is committed to addressing the needs of individuals with insurance who cannot afford their co-payments, co-insurance, insurance premiums, or other out-of-pocket healthcare costs. The specific amount of assistance for myeloma patients varies from year to year, as well as the period of time applications will be accepted.

Once the HealthWell Foundation budget for the year has been exhausted, the program is closed until the next calendar year. Applications for help should be submitted as soon after January 1 as possible.

www.healthwellfoundation.org
P.O. Box 4133
Gaithersburg, MD 20878
Phone: 800-675-8416
Fax: 800-282-7692

Leukemia and Lymphoma Society

The Leukemia and Lymphoma Society is dedicated to funding blood cancer research, education, and patient services. Its mission: Cure leukemia, lymphoma, and myeloma; and meanwhile, improve the quality of life of patients and their families. Their co-pay program helps patients meet their health insurance or Medicare Part B or D premiums or co-pay obligations. Currently, the maximum annual grant to myeloma patients is $10,000. Be certain your myeloma diagnosis is noted. Maximum grants to patients with other cancers may be less.

www.lls.org/copay
Information/Research Center, Phone: 800-955-4572
Co-Pay Assistance Program, Phone: 877-557-2672

Patient Access Network Foundation

The Patient Access Network Foundation provides financial support for out-of-pocket costs. These include deductible amounts, co-pays, co-insurance, costs of a wide range of drugs, and costs of other health conditions not directly linked to myeloma. This is an important subtlety, as it may bring side effects, health matters that relate in obscure ways, and independent, simultaneous health issues—called co-morbidities—under the coverage umbrella. It is currently offering myeloma patients who qualify up to $10,000 per year in assistance.

www.panfoundation.org
P.O. Box 221858
Charlotte, NC 28222
Phone: 866-316-PANF (7263)

Patient Advocate Foundation—and Its Fund—Patient Advocate Foundation Co-Pay Relief

Patient Advocate Foundation was founded in 1996 to help with specific problems patients may face with a health insurer over coverage and claims, or with an employer who takes steps against the best interests of a person due to a health condition. Clients are assigned a case manager who will direct them to valuable outside resources in their specific area of need.

In 2004, the Co-Pay Relief was founded to help patients with their out-of-pocket pharmaceutical expenses. Myeloma patients may receive up to $10,000 annually.

www.patientadvocate.org
Phone: 800-532-5274
www.copays.org
700 Thimble Shoals Blvd., Suite 200
Newport News, VA 23606
Phone: 866-512-3861
Fax: 757-873-8999

Tip #3—All the drug companies that matter to you offer ways to help defray the cost of using their products.

There are two sorts of programs to be aware of: direct help from the drug manufacturer, and help from an intermediary through a *patient assistance program.*

Drug Manufacturer Direct Help Programs

You can pretty well assume that the drugs prescribed for you are priced in the stratosphere and that despite all the programs and insurance and price negotiation that intercede, you can expect that some part of that unbelievable sum, waaay up there, will fall to earth and kick you in the wallet.

Start the process of seeking financial relief now. Get the list of drugs you're taking. Find out who the manufacturers are. Get on the phone or the Internet.

One other suggestion: You may not be poor; you may assume that your financial position will disqualify you for this sort of help. That may or may not be the case. Call the phone numbers listed here rather than going to the Internet address. Tell the service person who will eventually get on the line about your concern. Listen carefully. These qualification rules are sometimes largely gamesmanship: Play the game, get the discount.

Amgen
Drugs: Xgeva, Neupogen, Epogen, Neulasta
Amgen Reimbursement Connection
800-272-9376 | www.amgen.com/amgenassist/amgen_assist.html

Celgene
Drugs: Thalomid, Revlimid, and Pomalidomide
Celgene's Patient Support Solutions
800-931-8691 | www.celgenepsc.com

Centocor Ortho Biotech
Doxil Reimbursement Hotline 800-609-1083 | www.doxiline.com/doxiline/pages/patientassist/intro.jsp

Procrit Reimbursement Hotline 800-553-3851 | www.procritline.com

Genentech
Drug: Rituxan
Genentech Access Solutions 888-249-4918 | www.genentechaccesssolutions.com/portal/site/AS

Millennium
Drug: Velcade
Velcade Assistance Program 866-835-2233 | www.velcade.com/Paying-for-treatment

Novartis
Drugs: Aredia and Zometa
Novartis Patient Assistance Program 800-282-7630 | www.us.zometa.com/patient/zometa-reimbursment-help.jsp

Onyx Pharmaceuticals
Drug: Kyprolis
Onyx 360-855-669-9360 | www.onyx.com/therapies/patientaccess/onyx-360

Sanofi US
Drugs: Mozobil and Leukine
Journey Partners Program 800-981-2491 | www.sanofi.us

Patient Assistance Programs

When drug company-run assistance programs began, the forthright intent was to provide help directly to patients and their medical teams. As is so often the case in this convoluted world, matters became so complicated that thwarted patients turned to politicians, lawyers, social workers, and case nurses for help with the red tape.

The drug companies were equally frustrated, first by their genuine concerns for patient welfare, then by sometimes destructive legislation and conflicting state and federal agency mandates.

From this soil have sprung today's *patient assistance programs,* guides that point the way through the jungle.

Most provide their services at no cost to patients. Some help for a fee. Be cautious, most particularly if asked for an upfront fee. You have no enforceable guarantee that you will be satisfied by the outcome.

There are several websites that give information about patient assistance programs and may even provide you an application. It is important to be sure the site is up to date, as the programs frequently change.

Some of the better-known ones are described here.

RxAssist

RxAssist specializes in drug assistance programs for those who are disabled, have low incomes, or are Medicare beneficiaries. Included are programs that provide coverage for Medicare Part D beneficiaries who are having financial difficulty due to a gap in coverage.

www.rxassist.org
111 Brewster Street
Pawtucket, RI 02860
Phone: 401-729-3284
Fax: 401-729-2955

Needy Meds

Needy Meds is a source of information on *thousands* of programs that may be able to offer assistance to people in need. Needy Meds does not have an application, nor can it answer questions on individual assistance programs. It strives to provide accurate and current information, but asks that you contact specific programs directly with questions.

Needy Meds also offers a free drug discount card that may help you obtain a substantially lower price on your medications. This card can be used instead of insurance or by anyone without insurance.

www.needymeds.org
P.O. Box 219
Gloucester, MA 01931

Phone: 978-865-4115
Fax: 419-858-7221

The Partnership for Prescription Assistance

The Pharmaceutical Research and Manufacturer's Association, an advocate for the pharmaceutical industry, runs Partnership for Prescription Assistance. The program's mission is to increase awareness of patient assistance programs and to boost enrollment of those who are eligible. It offers a single point of access to more than 475 public and private programs, including nearly 200 offered by pharmaceutical companies.

www.pparx.org
Phone: 888-4PPA-NOW (477-2669)

Tip #4—You may get help with out-of-town medical travel.

CancerCare's Door to Door Program

This program provides individual grants up to $100/year to cancer patients of any type. In addition, multiple myeloma patients can receive up to $150 per quarter, $600/year, reimbursement for transportation costs such as gasoline, taxi, bus or train fare to and from a doctor's office. Patients must meet certain eligibility criteria and provide documentation such as receipts.

www.cancercare.org
800-813-HOPE (4673)

Public Benefit Flying

A series of well-meaning programs for giving cancer patients free flights to medical treatment have been around for years. The mode of travel is private aircraft, ranging in size from Piper Cub to corporate jet. When all the arrangements and requirements meld, this can be a wonderful way to get somewhere. Certainly, the private aircraft operators are delightful.

But:

- Unless you can hop aboard unaided and travel with little or no medical paraphernalia, you may not be able to get the ride.
- If you expect a wheelchair, oxygen, or some other medical amenity to be available, you'd best make certain or take your own.
- There may not be room for all the luggage you normally take. Both bulk and weight restrictions may apply.
- These are little planes. Most fly low and slow and sometimes bouncy. You may find this change from Boeing and Airbus lots of fun. Some people

discover that this sort of flying takes getting used to.

- Be sure you know what, if any, altitude restriction your doc places on you. The pilot may ask.
- Flights do not always keep to schedules and do not always take off or land where they are supposed to. You had better have Plan B at the ready, and room on a credit card for a last-minute commercial flight.
- These flights often begin or end at an airfield much smaller than you are used to. The normal amenities of commercial air may not be available. Parking may be wholly unattended and food service may be out of a vending machine.
- If you have an emergency medical need, the best help available may be the paramedic from a nearby fire station.
- The good news is that Homeland Security dictums are fewer. You can carry your open bottle of water and toenail clippers aboard. You miss the opportunity to stand in long lines while the contents of your luggage are being tossed and your naked profile is up on somebody's big-screen TV.

The Air Care Alliance

The Air Care Alliance is an umbrella organization for public benefit flying organizations. To get a ride, click on its website or phone the toll-free number. Choose an organization. Open a conversation.

www.aircareall.org/listings.htm
Phone: 888-260-9707

Free Places to Stay

American Cancer Society Hope Lodges

The American Cancer Society (ACS) offers cancer patients and their caregivers a free, temporary place to stay when their best hope for effective treatment may be in another city. Each Hope Lodge provides a nurturing, home-like environment where patients can relax in private rooms. Every Hope Lodge also offers a variety of resources and information about cancer and how best to fight the disease. There is access to the ACS's 24-hour toll-free call center and website, as well as a comprehensive on-site library designed to help patients and caregivers make informed decisions. There are currently 31 Hope Lodges in the United States.

www.cancer.org/treatment/supportprogramservices/hopelogde/hope-lodge-nationwide-supporters
Phone: 800-ACS-2345 (227-2345)

Joe's House

Joe's House is a nonprofit organization providing a nationwide online service that helps cancer patients and their families find lodging near treatment centers. Its mission is to centralize the various lodging options and to streamline the reservation process by listing various types of lodging throughout the United States that are close to hospitals and treatment centers. Details on each lodging facility are available with information on amenities, rates, and reservation methods and requirements. Joe's House works with these hotels and other lodging facilities to centralize inventory and provide medical discounts to cancer patients.

www.joeshouse.org
Phone: 877-JOESHOU (563-7468)

Healthcare Hospitality Network (Formerly known as The National Association of Hospital Hospitality Houses, Inc.)

This is another omnibus listing for lodging and other supportive services to patients and their families. Nationally, more than 150 members of the National Association of Hospital Hospitality Houses, Inc. (NAHHH) provide warm, caring support for over a quarter of a million people each year. NAHHH housing costs $5 to $15. Sometimes it's free. Many of its hospitality houses and inns are also listed on the Joe's House website.

www.nahhh.org
Phone: 800-542-9730

Other Free and Low-Cost Housing

A growing number of hospitals with myeloma teams have concierge services to meet the housing and other needs of out-of-town patients. Call the hospital's general information number. Ask for the hospitality help person, the concierge, or the hospital travel coordinator.

You may wonder why neither Burger King nor Ronald McDonald House charities are mentioned. These wonderful housing programs serve youthful patients only.

8

Myeloma Tax Savings: Minimize Your Tax Burden and Get Some Money Back

George Russell, CPA

Recordkeeping and attention to detail will pay off.

Some medical expenses lower the income taxes of some people. Not much to hang your hat on, I know, but as a CPA, hyperbole is frowned on. That said, as a guy with considerable experience helping cancer patients and their families get something back at tax time, I know I can save you money.

I must warn you that tax law is a highly effective sedative. You'll be able to follow it and learn, but you would have had more fun with your nose in a good novel. Just be patiently persistent. In a sense, searching tax law for benefits is like going through the cushions of an enormous sofa. Gems will be discovered. Also cookie crumbs. If you have a mindset that endures this sort of thing, join me. If not, take this chapter to your tax adviser. Armed with this knowledge, he or she will be able to arrange your tax affairs so that savings result.

General Income Guidelines

The tax code affords the most income adjustments to those with lower incomes. As a guideline, if you and your family report annual income of $150,000, you're going to need medical deductions that probably exceed $11,250 for the bottom line to be improved. If income is $50,000, medical expenses of $3,750 could make a worthwhile difference.

Overall, my suggestion is that—whatever the income—keep track of expenses and let your tax preparer sort out this complicated situation.

Qualified Expenses and How They Become Tax Deductions

The Internal Revenue Service uses the term *qualified medical expenses* and blames Congress for the controversy over which costs are acceptable versus which are not. Endless litigation and politicking have resulted, as you can imagine. But for the purpose of learning the ropes, please accept the fact that there is a list, and that all of a myeloma patient's medical expenses are probably on it.

Qualified medical expenses are the costs of diagnosis, cure, mitigation, treatment, or prevention of disease, and the costs for treatments affecting any part or function of the body. They include the costs of equipment, supplies, and diagnostic devices needed for these purposes. They also include dental and ophthalmological expenses.

Medical care expenses must be primarily to alleviate or prevent a physical or mental defect or illness. They do not include expenses that the IRS believes are merely beneficial to general health, such as vitamins and vacation—unless you have written doctor's orders. Then an examiner's sense that your claim is reasonable may permit it ... that's "may," not will.

Medical expenses include the premiums you pay for health insurance and the amounts you pay for transportation to get medical care. Medical expenses also include amounts paid for qualified long-term care services and limited amounts paid for any qualified long-term care insurance contract.

A Partial List of Acceptable Deductions

Alcoholism treatment	Fertility enhancement	Organ transplant
Ambulance	Guide dog/service animal	Oxygen
Artificial limb	Health insurance premiums	Physical examination
Artificial teeth	Hearing aid	Prosthesis
Autoette	Imaging	Psychiatric care
Bandage	Lab fee	Psychologist
Body scan	Legal fees to obtain treatment	Sterilization
Braille book and magazine	Lifetime care-advantage payments	Stop-smoking programs

Contact lens and supplies	Medical conferences	Surgery
Crutch	Medical equipment	Telephone equipment for the deaf
Dental treatment	Medical information plan	Therapy
Diagnostic device	Medical supplies	Vasectomy
Drug addiction treatment	Medicare premiums	Weight-loss program, prescribed
Eye surgery or keratotomy	Nursing home	Wheelchair
Eyeglasses	Nursing services	Wigs due to illness

Some Nondeductible Items: A Partial List of Unacceptable Deductions

Childcare, normal	Health club dues	Nonprescribed items for general health
Cosmetic surgery, elective	Illegal drugs	Swimming lessons
Dancing lessons	Life insurance	Teeth whitening
Funeral expenses	Medical care, future	Veterinary fees
Hair transplant		

Transportation

Cost of both local and out-of-town travel is deductible. Local travel can be calculated by a mileage allowance, 24 cents per mile starting January 1, 2013, or by adding up actual direct expenses such as gas and taxi fare. Parking fees and tolls are allowed in addition to mileage.

Out-of-town, travel includes air fare, bus fare, cab rides, meals, and so forth. Lodging that was necessary to receive treatment by a licensed medical provider can be deducted up to $50 per day. Be aware that if the place you stay offers especially nice recreation or vacation amenities, an examiner is apt to take a harder look at it.

Because of the debilitating nature of myeloma, a companion's reasonable travel costs—for both local and out-of-town medical treatment—in many cases is deductable.

Plastic Surgery

Cosmetic repair that is medically necessary, or that corrects deformities due to a medical condition, is deductible. An example of this is breast reconstruction after surgery.

Distinction Between Types of Drugs

What you paid for prescription medicines is deductible. The cost of medicines that do not require a prescription, such as aspirin, is not deductible even though doctor recommended. My personal advice is to obtain copies of prescriptions for all medicines even though not deductible.

Health Practitioners

Services of an acupuncturist, chiropractor, osteopath, optometrist, and Christian Science practitioner are deductible. Costs of other healers, both licensed and unlicensed, will probably not be questioned, but may be. Native American healing ceremonies have been allowed.

Home Improvements

Changes to your home may be deductible if made to accommodate a medical disability. Examples are: entrance or exit ramps; widening doorways and hallways; installing railings, support bars, or other modifications to bathrooms; lowering or modifying kitchen cabinets and equipment; moving or modifying electrical outlets and fixtures; installing porch and stair lifts; modifying fire alarms, smoke detectors, and other warning systems; modifying stairways; adding handrails or grab bars in bathrooms and elsewhere; modifying hardware on doors; modifying areas in front of entrance and exit doorways; and grading the ground to provide access to the residence.

These expenses are deductible only to the extent that they exceed the increase in value of the property. The IRS has a complex calculation to determine this amount. An elevator generally increases the property value and in spite of its high cost usually provides minimal deduction.

Long-Term Care

Long-term care facilities that are primarily necessary for medical reasons are also deductible. Other home care or homes for the elderly is not deductible, but costs of medical services and medicines provided while the taxpayer is there are deductible.

Qualified long-term care insurance premiums were deductible with the following limits as of 2013:

Age 40 or under—$360.
Age 41 to 50—$680.
Age 51 to 60—$1,360.
Age 61 to 70—$3,640.
Age 71 or over—$4,550.

Permutations

The full amount of medical expenses is not deductible. Congress, in its infinite wisdom, decided that some amount of medical expense is normal—which, for some reason, makes it not deductible. The floor of expenses that must be passed is 7 1/2% of *adjusted gross income* (AGI), a term that is quite precise. Please follow me closely: as one goes through the exercise of calculating tax obligation using the IRS standard long form (known as Form 1040), AGI is the total of amounts that precedes exemptions and itemized or standard deductions. AGI includes net rents, net business income, and net capital gains and losses.

AGI is the number shown on line 37 of 2012 Form 1040.

To receive any tax benefit From medical expenses, two thresholds must be passed. Because of the 7 1/2% floor, a return with AGI of $100,000 cannot include medical expenses in itemized deductions until medical expenses exceed $7,500, and includes only the amounts in excess of $7,500. The 7 1/2% floor increases to 10% for the tax years starting after 2012 for taxpayers under age 65.

Next, itemized deductions in total must exceed the taxpayer's standard deduction. The standard deduction varies based on the taxpayer age, blindness, and marital status. The standard deduction amount is indexed for inflation. Also, as AGI increases, the standard deduction is phased out. For 2013 a single person under age 65 claimed a standard deduction of $6,100; a married couple $12,200. The standard deduction for 2013 is increased $1,200 for each individual age 65 and above, and for each blind individual.

Planning Can Increase a Medical Expense Deduction

The 7 1/2% medical expense floor, the standard deduction, and itemized deduction rules present a planning opportunity. By lumping the medical expense payments and the payment of itemized deductions into one year and then taking the standard deduction in another year, you may be able to get more tax advantage from your medical expenses. You do this by making all your medical expense payments in one year's tax period.

Payments

Payment of medical expenses can be made by cash, check, pay-by-phone or online, or by credit card. Payments are deductible in the year paid, not the year of service.

Payment by check is credited for tax purposes on the day the check is mailed or delivered; pay-by-phone and online payments are credited on the date shown by the financial institution. Payment by credit card is official when the amount is charged, even if you pay your credit card bill years later.

Alternative Minimum Tax

In 1969, Congress decided that too many wealthy individuals were avoiding taxes by taking advantage of the tax planning allowances created by that august body in earlier years. The *alternative minimum tax* (AMT) was devised to rectify the situation. Inflation now causes the AMT to impact taxpayers with moderate income.

Taxpayers who are subject to the alternative minimum tax may also deduct medical expenses, but a 10% floor replaces the 7 1/2% floor discussed earlier.

The AMT exemption amounts for 2013 are $51,900 for a single taxpayer, and $80,800 for a joint return. As AGI increases, the exemption is phased out.

Payment Option Plans

Several types of accounts can be set up to pay medical expenses, with a variety of tax consequences. These accounts will be beneficial to limited numbers of taxpayers and the rules get quite complex. This discussion is general. Anyone establishing one of these accounts should review the rules carefully with his or her tax advisor.

Health Savings Account

A health savings account (HSA) allows a taxpayer to make contributions to a trust account. The contributions are deducted from AGI, so no deduction floor rules apply. Amounts are then withdrawn tax free to use to pay medical expenses. You receive no tax deduction upon paying the medical expenses. The deduction came when you contributed to the HSA.

An HSA can be set up if your only health insurance policy is a high-deductible health plan. Certain other coverage is permitted, such as accident, disability, dental, vision, and long-term care policies.

Medicare recipients do not qualify for HSAs.

In addition to high deductibles, these plans have out-of-pocket limits for 2013 were:

	Deductible	Out-of Pocket
	Minimum	Maximum
Self	$1,250	$6,350
Family	$2,500	$12,500

Archer Medical Savings

These plans are very similar to HSAs but could not be established after 2007. A taxpayer may still contribute to an existing Archer.

The Flexible Spending Arrangement (FSA)

Under an employer's IRC Section 125 cafeteria plan, a taxpayer may exclude a portion of income from tax by placing it into an FSA for health care. This tax-free money is then used to pay medical expenses. As this income was not taxed, no deduction is available when the expense is paid. The amount that can be contributed is limited by terms of the plan. Any part of the contribution not spent before year's end is lost, so careful planning is required

The Health Reimbursement Arrangements (HRAs)

This is another sort of plan set up by employers. Under an HRA, employees are reimbursed by their employers for the medical expenses they pay. The employee is not taxed on this reimbursement, nor does the employee deduct any expense. Reimbursement limits are set by the employer. The employer pays the medical expenses.

Caveat

Things in the tax world change. All the time. As do interpretations of existing rules, regulations, what's *fair,* and what are *usual practices.* We now spend about six billion hours a year complying with nearly four million words of federal tax code. For perspective, a billion hours ago, our ancestors lived in trees.

Caveat emptor.

9

Your Workplace: Myeloma Changes Everything

Sickness and treatment are new, permanent work conditions.

"I was playing tennis. I had just hit a high lob when I felt something snap in my chest. I went over to Little Company of Mary (hospital) and got a friend of mine in Radiation to take an x-ray. I'll never forget the look on his face when he came out with the film. 'Jim, you broke a rib. But that's not the worst of it...' and I couldn't get him to look me in the eye."

"That was the beginning of the end of my practice. Even though I wasn't ready to let the still, small voice in the back of my head be recognized, my life changed right there."

—Jim Tamkin, MD

The Impact of the News

The fact that you have myeloma will be riveting news to your co-workers. Some of them—perhaps all—will be emotionally devastated. They will also contemplate what losing your work skills will mean to the team. This is very high-powered stuff. Take charge of as much of the disclosure process as you can. Your co-workers, and maybe your boss, need your informed, level-headed crisis leadership.

Some of the news about your illness is already out there. It hit like a blast wave, shocking everyone. You or somebody in your inner circle is expected to explain the rest.

You should do that. Carefully and without joking: You need a two-part message. First, explain that you have a form of cancer that will lead to grave but not necessarily terminal illness; and second, tell them that you have decided upon a plan for transition from your present job to a life with less work and more time for treatment.

Be as positive and confident as possible. It creates the best environment for events that follow.

Each person's work situation is different. You must make the decisions that are right for you and your family.

You may find that you need to take a step back from work to focus on treatment. That may mean taking a leave of absence, reducing your hours, or leaving your job.

There is no right answer for everyone. Consider your options carefully, and understand the potential impact on your finances and your health coverage. Do what's best for you—not your work, not your employer. Be pointedly selfish.

Four principles to keep you on safer ground:

1. Don't lie.

2. Don't tell different people different things.

3. The briefer explanation is usually better for you than the longer one.

4. If an employee assistance professional (EAP), as discussed a little further on, is available, seek that person's counsel on this entire matter.

Consider Opening a Facebook or Caring Bridge Page

You or someone close to you knows how to open Facebook or to find a website called Caring Bridge. You can put your story and any general messages you have for those who know you on one of these billboards. Facebook is very public and easy to find. Caring Bridge gives access to those who know you while keeping out the riffraff.

Have an Answer to "What Can I Do?"

You need things now. You'll need others later. A personal page that people with computers can go to without bothering you is a good place for you, your caregiver, and family to brief those who know you and to keep them up to date on your progress.

Don't tell people there's nothing they can do for you, even if it's true. Have a need or two in mind or refer those who ask to your computer page. At least two ways to be helpful can always be suggested: prayer and a donation in your name to a myeloma-fighting nonprofit charity.

Prayer in the Co-Worker Context

Work is a secular place. Broad religious divergence is to be expected. You yourself may not practice any sort of observance. It is still befitting your new circumstance to ask people to pray for you, or to keep you in their thoughts.

Employee Assistance Professionals Help

A majority of U.S. organizations have an EAP available. This person is your advocate, in place to guide you through myeloma's impact on your job and on your employer. Your EAP is also there as coach, so that you take maximum advantage of health benefits and sickness provisions.

This person is not beholden to the HR department. Your condition—really anything you say to your EAP—goes no further without your express permission.

Marina London, the spokesperson for the EAP Association, suggests that if you work for an organization without an EAP, seek the counsel of a hospital social worker.

The EAP of a spouse can also serve you.

"Many of us are licensed clinical social workers (LCSW), as well as certified employee assistance professionals (CEAP)," London, who holds both credentials, says. "We've helped in these situations many times: finding a good support group, locating child and elder care, guiding a person through the provisions of the Americans with Disabilities Act, budget and credit counseling. EA professionals are experts in short-term solutions. When one works with an expert who knows the topography, more gets done in less time."

Other Resources

"The American Cancer Society and the International Myeloma Foundation also offer free, expert counseling," reminds London. "You may also benefit by visiting www.patientslikeme.com. Two MIT engineers started it. 170,000 patients with100,000 different sorts of illness offer experiences and wisdom."

Forecasting the Bumpy Road Ahead

Myeloma is a general condition that does not progress in the same way or at the same speed from one patient to the next. Various treatment plans add to the complexity of figuring out how a person will fare in years ahead. It is not all gloom and doom, as it was until very recently. Today's treatment protocols frequently lead to extended remissions.

Help with Forecasting

"There are clinicians we know who specialize in helping people plan their way through the rest of their lives," London says. "Most patients have health insurance resources that will pay for this valuable insight."

10

Looking Ahead: Estate and Practical Planning

Malin Dollinger, MD, FACP

Sign on the front lawn of a Great Bend funeral home: Drive carefully. We'll wait.

A Fragile Hope Considered

Recent improvements in treatment allow myeloma patients to continue quality lives for much longer than ever before. Cruel as it is to offer a hope that may not materialize, some myeloma patients—no one knows which—will live for many years, possibly until the means is found to stop or even reverse the course of this cancer.

Especially since there is new hope, it makes sense to consider and to prepare for predictable events.

Living with Mortality: Life Goes On

Though we all know deep down that we are mortal and that our lives will end, it's the American way to block out the lesson that other people, whose deaths were the furthest things from their minds, teach us daily by their passing. Now we face myeloma and the certainty that mortality is not a *sometime,* and may possibly be a *soon.* We find ourselves in a strange and upsetting frame of mind that considers living and dying at the same time.

How can we cope? Can we adjust to it and renew our interest in life's goals and pleasures? Is it better not to look too openly at this illness, and perhaps deny its likely outcome? After all, experts have been wrong before.

In the 50 years since I graduated from Yale's medical school, I have counseled a great many cancer patients. I have learned to believe in hope and sometimes hope rewards me. But beyond hope is mortality, which is a certainty. We're all going to die of something, sometime. It seems logical to use the presence of myeloma as a springboard to actions we should have taken anyway.

Matters Deserving Your Attention

Faith

The contributors to this chapter are all men and women of faith, both Jews and Christians. We have prayed for you and for each other. We do not mean to proselytize. But we want you to be aware of our strongly held, unanimous opinion on this subject.

Beyond that—and this is the nut of it—there is conclusive evidence that men and women of faith cope more successfully in extreme environments, such as when one faces the conditions and stresses that come with myeloma.

I suggest to those readers who have a faith, that it be held close. Or, if it has not been examined recently, that it be renewed.

Forgiveness

Have you been grievously wronged? Is there someone you absolutely cannot abide? Hate can be tasty, even sustaining, but it can't be healing. Forgiveness can make you well and give you peace.

Is there something you have done that you have never forgiven yourself for? Forgiveness does not permit forgetfulness, nor does it pardon the cost. But it takes away your role as a punisher.

As your doctor—at least through the end of this chapter—consider this a prescription: Forgive others, and forgive yourself.

Prepare and Implement an Advance Directive

You are ill and need a considerable amount of medical attention. Should circumstances cause your health to deteriorate to a point where you remain alive but cannot return to what *you* consider a decent quality of life, the men and women caring for you need to be told what you want them to do. A tool of law called an *advance directive* serves this purpose.

"The sick person has to start the awkward conversation," advises Fred Corbalis, a family law attorney at Spierer and Woodward, LLC, Redondo Beach, California. "It is very hard for others to talk to a loved one about treatment options affecting life and death." He suggests a first exploration of the subject with the patient's physician. In a worst-case scenario, what things may happen? What happens then? As details and consequences are explained by a trusted medical expert, the matters that should be covered in an advance directive become clear. Corbalis suggests a follow-up meeting with a qualified family law attorney. We live in an increasingly contentious world. "Many hospitals hope to see advance directives on law firm stationery," he says.

Having created the advance directive, consider its impact on those who love you. "I would also suggest that the administration of the directive be put into the hands of someone who can make decisions and not be haunted by the consequences," says Corbalis. In particular, bedside decisions about life or death are inhumane to force on spouses, he says. A member of the patient's clergy might be one choice. The family doctor is another.

In my own practice, when speaking with the family of the grievously ill, I will say, "Of course you know (the patient) very well. Imagine that he/she were standing here with us, knowing what we know about the situation. What do you think he/she would counsel us to do?" I could expect a fair answer that we would all be comfortable with, and that would be guilt-free.

Corbalis also suggests that several copies of the advance directive be put in the hands of those who may need to be guided by it. Include the local hospital and the patient's primary oncologist.

The contents of an advance directive should not be secret, Corbalis says. Family and friends should know the decisions that have been made so that no one tries to steer matters in a direction the patient doesn't want.

An advance directive probably won't cost a lot. A meeting of less than an hour in an attorney's office should be sufficient.

An advance directive can also be developed with the help of the patient's primary care physician, clergy, or the qualified person on staff at a hospital.

Your Will

Next in order of importance is your last will and testament. Like your advance directive, it must be prepared with careful, sober consideration for the well-being of those you love, and be completed before any sense that death is imminent distorts the matter.

To digress for just a moment, we sometimes hear about some disgruntled person "'breaking"' a will to get a share of the estate. In fact, that almost never happens when the document is prepared by an attorney, Corbalis says. So, for purposes of this discussion, we won't go into how a will is best constructed. We shall presume that the will was prepared by an attorney and that it will fulfill its mission.

We shall also presume that it fairly and properly passes along your worldly possessions. Our intent is to encourage you to make certain that this important matter is taken care of, not to make suggestions about what should go to Niece Jenny.

Here are six principles to consider when planning a will:

1. The preparation of a will is an act of compassion. Clearly and carefully give your possessions to those you have in mind and to those who are positioned to continue processes you care about, on your behalf.

2. Don't use your will as a weapon.

3. Don't reward greed.

4. When your will is done, consider its effect on those you will leave behind, the business and

other institutions it may affect, and your community. Hope for the good your gifts may do.

5. If you can do it, tell beneficiaries what has been decided face-to-face, rather than through an executor. High expectations and a contentious family atmosphere are the two most common complicating factors. Both lose much of their power to disrupt when the will is well-established public knowledge.

6. Those who die without a will leave the task of sorting out their affairs to the state they lived in. A state appointee, using court-established guidelines, becomes responsible. The only circumstance in which this may be satisfactory is when the person died penniless and without possessions.

Debt and Asset Management

There are all sorts of special circumstances that require some thought as we approach the end of days. Some of us live comfortably ... in homes with hundreds of thousands of dollars of mortgage debt. A huge payout to the mortgage holder can be a problem during estate settlement proceedings.

Some of us own family businesses, like farms, that are going to become estate taxable assets. They may have to be sold, maybe in a steeply discounted fire sale, to pay Uncle Sam and the governor. Other valuables that enrich the lives of family members may also end up in the tax collector's crosshairs.

Those who understand these matters assure me that these predicaments may not be impossible to overcome. My point to you is that these matters should be faced while there is time for creative solutions to be considered. A financial adviser, a CPA, or an attorney will be able to guide you.

When the End of Life Is in Sight

"In 1959, it was discovered by Leonard Hayflick and Paul Moorehead that normal cells in our bodies will only divide a fixed number of times. It is believed that each cell has its own 'death clock' ... This theory is called the Hayflick limit."

—Josefa Azcueta, RN, OCN

A Clear and Simple Vision

It seems to me that being advised of death's approach lifts a great burden from a person. There is no longer any pressure to aspire. You've made it. You are where you are...' round the bases and safe at home plate, so to speak. The vision is clear and simple. Complications have fallen away. What remains is for any resolution that honor or good sense demand.

For many people, hope remains as well. It is, after all, in our DNA. It adds to the quality of the life we have left. And one *never* knows ... significant numbers of cancer patients recover from near death. Richard Bloch, the "R" in H & R Block, lived 14 years after the best minds in oncology gave him 3 months. His widow, Annette, and the R.A. Bloch Cancer Foundation, continue.

One of the most famous commentaries on this subject was by Winston Churchill, who glared at the boys of his alma mater, Harrow School, October 29, 1941, and said, "Never give in, never give in, never, never, never, never—in nothing great or small, large or petty—never give in, except to convictions of honor and good sense."

Hospice

There are many events in the health of a myeloma patient. Some are victories over conditions. Some require concessions, often accompanied by modified treatment strategy. Over time, myeloma gains ground. Over time, damage caused by disease, drugs, other treatments, surgeries—or all of them—bring the patient to a place that clearly signals the ebb of life. Quite often the patient is the first to understand. In fortunate circumstances, family and close friends come to the same knowledge at about the same time.

After the situation is acknowledged, the process of preparing for death begins.

Most commonly, the patient's doctor brings up hospice. Should that not happen, it is quite acceptable for the patient to ask for it.

Hospice focuses on treating symptoms, providing comfort, and maintaining dignity, instead of a succession of now-futile treatment pathways, which now do more harm than good. It is also the process by which the patient is sheltered from the harshness that myeloma brought to its victims before this modern era. Hospice offers an almost cost-free accommodation to patient and family. All needs, from drugs and medical care to legal services, hospital equipment, and counseling are provided.

Hospice programs are available for hospitalized patients and those who decide to stay at home. Sometimes physical conditions require a hospital stay, but usually the patient may choose.

The new team of doctors and nurses that provide hospice care are trained to help the patient continue life as normally as possible, free of most discomforts and of unnecessary physical limitations. Beyond these generalities, hospice becomes highly personalized, providing comfort, security, and serenity on the patient's terms.

HOSPICE

HOPE

OPPORTUNITY

SERENITY

PEACE

INSPIRATION

COMFORT

EQUANIMITY

Part Three

Managing Treatment

11

Humuhumunukunukuapuaa*: Things to Know about Your Drugs

[* Per Harry Owens's Royal Hawaiians on 1960s TV: "I want to go back to my little grass shack in Kealakekua Hawaii/Where the OO-moo-HOO-moo-NOO-koo-NOO-koo-AH-poo-AH-ah goes swimming by...." "My Little Grass Shack in Kealakekua Hawaii," © 1933, lyrics and music by: Bill Cogswell, Tommy Harrison, and Johnny Noble.]

Dave Visel

The drugs you will take, what they are intended to do for you, and how they got those godawful names.

When I was a boy, we lived on a ranch outside Anaheim, California. Small by today's standards: just a house and barn and 10 acres of orange trees. Every so often, some trucks from our growers co-op, Sunkist, would pull up and out would pour a horde of pickers, jabbering in a language I could not understand.

My father told me it was Spanish. He said it was easy to learn if I just showed an interest. Sure enough, those guys taught me all sorts of things.

Later I became aware that much of what I had learned was best not used around my mother and that some of it required a greater understanding of human sexuality than I had at the time. But I digress.

My point is that new language may seem baffling at first, but with the help of people around you and a little practice, you can do fine. My further point is that, as a myeloma patient, this new language and the subjects it describes are not matters you have the luxury of ignoring.

A Similarity Between People in Lab Coats and Migrant Workers

The world of myeloma treatment features confounding new language that is, in my opinion, no more English than the words I learned in our orange grove: Methylprednisolone. Lenalidomide. Autologous. Cytogenetic. But here we are. And of course, we've got to learn enough to get along with the pickers.

Based on my own struggles with medical lingo, I suggest we begin by an examination of how these new terms are created and of how the names themselves become tools to our greater understanding of what's going on.

The Rules for Naming Drugs, Diseases, and Procedures

According to Wikipedia, the longest word in English has 189,816 letters.[5] It is the chemical name of titin, the largest protein molecule known. This and other names for organic chemical compounds have been derived by following six basic rules. To oversimplify a matter that desperately deserves it, an organic molecule's discoverer names the molecule's distinguishing feature, then attaches set, Latin-derived phrases that describe the molecule's other parts. When the name has been properly constructed in this way, other chemists, pharmacists, and treatment professionals have a good sense of what it is.

A similar process is used to name afflictions. Pneumonoultramicroscopic silicovolcanokoniosis, at a mere 45 letters, is an example. It is the longest word found in major dictionaries and describes a lung disease caused by the inhalation of very fine silica, leading to inflammation in the lungs. More simply, a

---

5 Methionylthreonylthreonylglutaminylarginyl ... isoleucine.

type of silicosis common in Hawaii, caused by inhaling volcanic dust.

So the stuff you hear in medical meetings is a construct of familiar terms and physical elements, strung together using set rules—like pig Latin (igpayatinlay). All you need to be completely conversant with what they're saying is a course in organic chemistry and some grasp of a language spoken in Rome 2,000 years ago.

First Rule of Language Management

Patients and their caregivers do a better job of managing their side of the street if they avoid in-depth medical education. Learn how to pronounce the terms. Learn at a practical level what each describes and why it should or shouldn't be part of your treatment.

Then apply this superficial medical knowledge to the areas that are important to health insurance management and maybe clinical trial participation; any disruptions to work or social obligations that the treatment may bring; any change in your physical abilities or appearance; and obligations that may have been neglected, such as the writing of an advance directive. Also, very importantly, don't leave those you know and love out of any of this. Discuss what you've learned with them to as full an extent as their attention spans will allow.

Whose Drugs Can You Trust?

We live in an era that distrusts doctors. And in the same breath with expressed cynicism about the medical community, people will blindly accept the healing claims of foods and herbs offered by health product retailers—even though few of these substances' uses are supported by any scientific evidence of effectiveness. This is a more or less innocent sport so long as general health, minor pain relief, and weight control are the sorts of objectives the consumer has in mind.

It is no longer harmless when the consumer's objective is to fight chronic disease. "I hold the health food and herb purveyors to the same standard as the pharmaceutical manufacturers," advises Daniel Lieber, MD, oncologist and hematologist, Angeles Clinic, Santa Monica, California. "If it has scientific evidence I can examine, I am pleased to invite the product into my practice." Dr. Lieber goes on to say that other, unsubstantiated remedies that can appear to be beneficial may not be good for you. With few exceptions, he and his colleagues simply don't have all the facts and can only hope for the best when facing patients who take them.

Dr. Lieber will also tell you that the drugs made by the pharmaceutical industry and approved by the Food and Drug Administration (FDA) for the treatment of myeloma patients—while better than ever—also have drawbacks. Nothing works all the time, or exactly as anticipated. It's just that when you are given drugs that have proven themselves after many millions of dollars of development and testing, the odds of the drug being helpful to you are better.

Life science companies today are among America's premier innovators. Six of the top 10 companies in global research and development expenditure are biopharmaceutical (the branch of pharmaceutical science that develops notable myeloma drugs), according to a 2010 report by Booz & Co.

"The biopharmaceutical industry's scientists have produced a global revolution in health care," says Kenneth C. Frazier, chief executive of Merck & Co., a leading manufacturer of drugs for myeloma. He adds that U.S. companies, including his own, account for 82% of the biotechnology research and development in the world, with more than 2,900 new medicines in the development pipeline.

Drugs Myeloma Patients Take

According to a current study, 1,240 drugs have been recently prescribed for patients with multiple myeloma. To save you from palpitations, this is not a list you are going to have to memorize. Nor will you have to take them all. The length of the list and the complexity of the pharmaceutical stew do illustrate the confounding nature of your disease and the number of twists and turns that its treatment may take. It is also fair to note that the list includes quite a number of compounds that duplicate the benefits of others on the list, or replace them.

Families of Drugs that Defeat Myeloma

Your medical team has chemical tools that perform various exotic jobs. They're all new. All promising. Also all experimental and never certain to provide the result you hope for.

Unless you have been steeped in medical science, you will find this whole families-of-drugs section a tough read, best waded through with access to the Internet or an oncology professional nearby. Don't—whatever you do—try to memorize this section. Just know that information about very powerful drug protocols is here. When you come to a point in your treatment when your oncologist tells you that you will begin receiving a *proteasome inhibitor* or that your new chemo features a *monoclonal antibody,* this section may help.

Visit the TBA Foundation website, www.tbafoundatio n.org, for more information on drugs.

Alkylating Agents

A class of drugs that kill cancer cells directly. They are, to use the medical term, cytotoxic. These guys also kill hair follicles. Some or all of your hair is going to fall out as a side effect of using these drugs.

Anthracycline Antibiotics

The anthracyclines are among the most effective anticancer treatments ever developed. But they are very hard on your heart. Your oncologist may put you on an anthracycline antibiotic for a limited time, during which a cardiologist will also be monitoring you.

Corticosteroids

All myeloma patients take these compounds periodically. They shrink tumors, also called plasmacytomas, which reduces pain.

Corticosteroids also reduce hypercalcemia (too much calcium in the blood). This eases constipation, nausea, stomach pain, poor appetite, and vomiting. Kidney pain is reduced and kidney stones are less likely to form. Frequent thirst and the need to urinate all the time are relieved.

The famous downsides are that you won’t rest well and you are apt to feel on edge. Weight gain and leg swelling also accompany use.

Bisphosphonates

Your disease attacks bone structure. Bisphosphonates protect it, reducing the risk of breaking a bone. Painful tumors in the bone, called lesions, are also reduced.

You will probably take either Zometa or Aredia, wonderfully effective drugs. You will be carefully monitored because bone loss in the jaw, osteonecrosis, may result. Kidney damage is also possible.

Growth Factors

Some of the drug families we discuss here are also called *growth factors.*

- Some encourage immature cells to become a specific sort of mature cell; a stem cell to become a white blood cell, for example.
- Others stimulate cell growth and division and are also referred to as *colony stimulating factors.*
- Some stop the growth of cells and may cause them to die.

Growth factor may be one of several uses for the drug. So when they say you're getting a growth factor, the proper reply is, *Which one?,* possibly followed by, *So, what is the objective?*

Growth Blockers

These drugs are designed to block the growth of myeloma cells by depriving them of substances they need, such as *vascular endothelial growth factor,* which you may hear referred to as VEGF. When tumor cells spread through the body, they release VEGF to create new blood vessels through a process known as angiogenesis (*angio*—blood vessel, *genesis*—creation). These blood vessels supply oxygen, minerals, and other nutrients to help cancer tumors grow, which is of course a bad thing.

Here are the 10 most common growth blockers used in myeloma therapy. Each is named after the type of chemical it blocks or inhibits.

1. Immunomodulators (often called IMiDs): Three drugs in this class are used when multiple myeloma has returned after remission. They are thalidomide (Thalomid), lenalidomide (Revlimid), and pomalidomide (Pomalyst). These medications stop the growth of blood vessels that feed tumors. They also boost the immune system and may kill cancer cells directly.

2. Proteasome inhibitors: Bortezomib (Velcade) was the first in its class of proteasome inhibitors, drugs that block the action of proteasomes, which are cellular complexes that break down proteins. Another promising drug, carfilzomib (Kyprolis), appears to work the same way as bortezomib and may be more effective for some patients.

3. Monoclonal antibodies: Often compared to guided missiles, monoclonal antibodies zero in on cancer cells whose surfaces have a target molecule. For example, the combination of lenalidomide

(Revlimid),[6] with a monoclonal antibody called elotuzumab (no brand name), holds promise in treating *refractory* multiple myeloma; that is, myeloma that comes back after it had disappeared for a time.

4. Histone deacetylase (HDAC) inhibitors: This class of drugs works by killing cancer cells or by stopping their growth. Two HDAC inhibitors, vorinostat (Zolinza), and panobinostat, a new drug that Novartis has not yet given a brand name, may be combined with proteasome inhibitors to help people whose tumors resist treatment with the proteasome inhibitor alone.

Name Your Poison

1950—Thalidomide is widely prescribed as a sedative and antimorning sickness drug during pregnancy.

1961—A study is published in *The Lancet,* a British medical journal, reporting that nearly 20% of women taking the drug deliver babies with severe abnormalities. More than 10,000 infants are affected.

1971—Judah Folkman, MD, publishes his hypothesis that thalidomide denies nutrition to cancerous

6 The scientific names for drugs discussed in this section are followed by their brand names in parenthese. Medical professionals will use either name, or both, without explanation. Our apologies for the confusion this creates. In case you wonder, it bewilders us as well.

tumors. The drug gains new respectability as an IMiD that is now prescribed for many myeloma patients.

—Excerpt, *From Infamy to Therapy,* Children's Hospital Boston, October 26, 2010

5. Akt (alkylphospholipids) inhibitor: An alkylphospholipids inhibitor disrupts cancer cell membranes and blocks the actions of proteins involved in cancer growth. An Akt inhibitor called perifosine (no brand name) holds promise as a treatment for multiple myeloma, when combined with bortezomib.

6. Heat shock protein (HSP)-90 inhibitors: HSPs are a class of functionally related proteins involved in the folding and unfolding of other protein molecules. They expand when exposed to elevated temperatures or other stress.

   Multiple myeloma cells contain more of an HSP, called Hsp90, than normal cells. The 90 refers to the protein's weight in kilodaltons. One dalton equals 1/12th of the weight of a radioactive carbon atom. A kilodalton is one thousand of them.

   Two drugs—alvespimycin (no brand name) and tanespimycin (whose developer, Bristol-Myers Squibb, may have given up on it)—block the actions of Hsp90. Research suggests that combining either of these drugs with bortezomib (Velcade) may be more effective than treatment with bortezomib alone.

7. Mammalian target of rapamycin (mTOR) inhibitors: This class of drugs blocks a mechanism called the mTOR pathway, which promotes tumor growth. Preliminary research suggests that combining lenalidomide (Revlimid) with an mTOR inhibitor called everolimus (Afinitor) may stall the growth of multiple myeloma.
8. Cyclin-dependent kinase (CDK) inhibitors: CDK inhibitors, such as the Chinese drug flavopiridol (Alvocidib) block proteins that promote the growth of multiple myeloma cells.
9. RANK ligand inhibitors: This new class of drugs is designed to block a factor in bone development known as RANK ligand. RANK ligand stimulates cells that break bone down. By blocking RANK ligand, these drugs increase bone density and strength. Denosumab (Xgeva), which is still experimental but promising, may be suggested if you have bones that need it.
10. Telomerase inhibitors: One drug, known as imetelstat (no brand name) blocks an important enzyme found to be active in 12 myeloma cell configurations. This enzyme allows cancer cells to resist chemotherapy.

"The first mention of a paid experimental subject comes from diarist Samuel Pepys, in an entry for November 21, 1667. He noted that the local college had hired a poor and debauched man to have some sheep blood let into his body. Although there had been plenty of consternation beforehand, the man apparently suffered no ill effects."

—John P. Bull, "The Historical Development of Clinical Therapeutic Trials"

Drugs in Clinical Trial

Every drug prescribed for a myeloma patient today is either going through, or has completed the clinical trial process. If all other factors are equal, minimize your risk by taking the medicine that has progressed through the clinical trial process the furthest or graduated from its clinical trial the longest time ago. It has more history out on the myeloma battlefield.

The development of a new drug begins in the lab and progresses to animal studies. If it passes very stringent examination and remains promising, it is tried out on a few volunteers (usually less than 100. This, a phase I clinical trial, is largely to measure safety. It is possible for a myeloma patient in dire need of the hoped-for benefit to participate in a phase I study, but it is ill advised except in a case where the patient has nothing to lose. This would be the pharmaceutical equivalent of the "Hail Mary pass" in football.

There are also phase I tests for drugs that have served patients with other medical conditions—just not myeloma. The drug's manufacturer and the FDA put it through this early testing process again because the drug is facing a new set of conditions. It is fair to presume that participating in this type of phase I testing is safer, but you should ask.

A larger group of patients participates in phase II development, which focuses on efficacy. Phase II testing may continue for months or years until all questions about the drug have been asked and answered by the drug developer and the FDA. Phase II studies often include a group of patients who get something other than the new medicine; this is often called the *control group.* They may get a dummy medicine called a *placebo,* or maybe an older drug that is considered effective, and whose results will be compared to outcomes among those testing the new brew.

> If you choose to participate in a clinical trial, you have the right to know if there is a control group and what medicine its members will be given.

Phase III clinical trials cap the development process. Hundreds to thousands of patients are involved. Myeloma and other blood cancer patients may be combined. By this point in the development process, the effectiveness of the drug is fairly certain. The purpose of the continued testing may be to compare its patient benefit or side effects to those of other medicines already in use.

A phase IV study—one or several—may follow, to answer the what-ifs that scientific nit-pickers are notorious for postulating. To make up something just for the purpose of illustration, a statistician might notice a possible variation in reaction among people with red hair, or among sailors, or overweight men. A special phase IV study could follow. The work done in this late phase research can be very valuable.

Off-Label Drug Uses

After a drug has made it through the clinical trial process, the FDA certifies it for the very specific uses studied during its testing. Those uses are then listed on the medicine's label or package insert and—please make special note—written in the journals of the insurance regulators who decide which drug therapies will be paid for and which will not.

Myeloma patients are members of a community representing about 1% of all cancer patients. There are drugs that have been developed for the other 99%, and for other diseases, that have interesting virtues. The doctors treating myeloma are constantly looking over the fence at the larger inventory of tools arrayed for other purposes and wondering if this one or that one might be just right for you. The difficulties are two: first, the doctor who chooses a drug for a use that has not been approved by the FDA—a use that is not on the drug's label—must take the drug through a qualification process. It may be simple and short, or it may require more steps and time, perhaps as much as a new clinical trial.

The second difficulty is that insurance companies may resist paying for off-label applications. You, the patient, should make certain that your medical team is also qualifying your new off-label treatment for insurance coverage.

Your drugs often cost hundreds to thousands of dollars per dose. Your medical team is rightly focused on result, not cost. Should you or your medical team's administrator fail to get payment approval from your insurance company before you receive the treatment, you may become obligated to pay this bill.

Drugs You May Be Given

These are the stars of the game. You may want to mark this page so that you can come back to it for reference. (Some of these compounds had not been given brand names at the time we went to press. Others will fail their trials or be replaced so you'll never see them again.)

Brand Name	Generic Name	Drug Class	FDA Approved
Adriamycin	doxorubicin	Anthracycline antibiotic	August 1974
Afinitor	everolimus	mTOR inhibitor	Phase III Clinical trial
Alkeran	melphalan	Alkylating agent	January 1964
Alvocidib	flavopiridol	CDK inhibitor	Phase I/II clinical trial
	dinaciclib	CDK inhibitor	Phase I/II clinical trial
Aplidin	plitidepsin	Antitumor agent	Phase III Clinical trial
	noscapine	Nonopiate alkaloid	Phase I Clinical trial
Aredia	pamidronate disodium	Bisphosphonate	October 1991
Bexxar	tositumomab	Monoclonal antibody	Phase II Clinical trial
Cytoxan	cyclophosphamide	Alkylating agent	November 1959
Decadron	dexamethasone	Corticosteroid	October 1958
Deltasone	prednisone	Corticosteroid	June 1955
Doxil	liposomal doxorubicin	Anthracycline antibiotic	November 1995
Epogen	erythropoietin	Colony stimulating factor	June 1989
Erivedge	vismodegib	Hedgehog inhibitor	Phase I Clinical trial
	enzastaurin	PKC inhibitor	Phase I Clinical trial
	masitinib	TK inhibitor	Phase III Clinical trial
HuMax	daratumumab	Monoclonal antibody	Phase I/II clinical trial

Brand Name	Generic Name	Drug Class	FDA Approved
	elotuzumab	Monoclonal antibody	Phase III Clinical trial
	siltuximab	Monoclonal antibody	Phase II Clinical trial
	mapatumumab	Monoclonal antibody	Phase I Clinical trial
	milatuzumab	Monoclonal antibody	Phase I/II clinical trial
	tabalumab	Monoclonal antibody	Phase I Clinical trial
	lorvotuzumab mertanisne	Monoclonal antibody	Phase I Clinical trial
Istodax	romidepsin	HDAC inhibitor	Phase II Clinical trial
Kyprolis	carfilzomib	Proteasome inhibitor	July 2012
	ixazomib	Proteasome inhibitor	Phase III Clinical trial
	delanzomib	Proteasome inhibitor	Phase I Clinical trial
	oprozomib	Proteasome inhibitor	Phase I Clinical trial
	marizomib	Proteasome inhibitor	Phase I Clinical trial
Medrol	methylprednisolone	Corticosteroid	October 1957
Mozobil	plerixafor	Stem cell mobilizer	December 2008
Neulasta	pegfilgrastim	Colony stimulating factor	January 2002
Neupogen	filgrastim	Colony stimulating factor	February 1991
Oncovin	vincristine	Alkylating agent	July 1963

Brand Name	Generic Name	Drug Class	FDA Approved
Pomalyst	pomalidomide	Immunomodulating agent	February 2013
Procrit	epoetin	Colony stimulating factor	June 1989
Revlimid	lenalidomide	Immunomodulating agent	June 2006
Sprycel	dasatinib	RTK inhibitor	Phase I/II clinical trial
Sutent	sunitinib	RTK inhibitor	Phase II Clinical trial
	obatoclax	Bcl-2 inhibitor	Phase I Clinical trial
	ibrutinib	BTK inhibitor	Phase I/II clinical trial
	dovitinib	FGFR inhibitor	Phase I Clinical trial
Thalomid	thalidomide	Immunomodulating agent	May 2006
Torisel	temsirolimus	mTOR inhibitor	Phase I/II clinical trial
Velcade	bortezomib	Proteasome inhibitor	May 2008
Xgeva	denosumab	RANK ligand inhibitor	Phase II/III clinical trial
	imetelstat	Telomerase inhibitor	Phase II Clinical trial
Zolinza	vorinostat	HDAC inhibitor	Phase III Clinical trial
	panobinostat	HDAC inhibitor	Phase III Clinical trial
	rocolinostat	HDAC inhibitor	Phase I Clinical trial
	perifosine	Akt inhibitor	Phase III Clinical trial (Halted)
	alvespimycin	Hsp90 inhibitor	Phase III Clinical trial

Brand Name	Generic Name	Drug Class	FDA Approved
	tanespimycin	Hsp90 inhibitor	Phase III Clinical trial (halted)
	AUY922	Hsp90 inhibitor	Phase I/II clinical trial
	ganetespib	Hsp90 inhibitor	Phase I clinical trial
Zometa	zoledronic acid	Bisphosphonate	August 2001

Your Treatment

Think of fighting myeloma as like fighting a major fire. You look to see what's burning. You bring water and whatever tools you think you need to the site as quickly as possible. You start to douse it, or clear-cut around it, or take some other measure that is more urgent to stop its progress. You get all the help you can. You constantly reassess what you're doing, paying particular attention to new outbreaks, shifts in the wind, sudden explosions, and the host of other surprises a fire can throw at you.

Drugs are tools that every myeloma treatment team has in hand, all the time. They are used in the context of current conditions, how the drug will work now, and how that work figures into the larger picture of the overall fight.

Damage is also a consideration. The disease causes damage. Sometimes the drugs do, too. Sometimes the drugs do far more than damage. They can disable or even threaten the life of the patient. Think back to the analogy of the fight against a major fire. There are circumstances in which one has to accept loss to gain a greater victory. There may be better tools—somewhere, sometime—but this is what you've got, and now is when something has to be done. You take your best shot, or you don't.

We grew up in the wealthiest, safest place of all time, with more accommodation and fewer inconveniences than any previous generation in the history of the planet has enjoyed. So thinking about danger and damage seems outrageous. Being in a battle, striking and receiving blows, is so out of the realm of our previous experience that some patients refuse to acknowledge what they face. For them, this fight is over. It never started. They pass from us rather quickly, comforted as best their doctors and families can.

> So, would you rather be a blindfolded passenger in the back seat, or see where you're going?

If you choose to fight, know as much as possible about the weapons available to you and how they are used. Also understand that nobody gets off the fire line unscathed.

The Piper Will Be Paid

It is safe to presume that any drug you are prescribed has been carefully selected to fight myeloma or some other condition that has shown up. But nothing in this fight is simple. You can almost bet that there will be a downside to any drug you take.

The Most Commonly Prescribed Drugs and Their Potential Side Effects

Brand name is followed by generic name.

Drug	Potential Side Effects
Decadron (dexamethasone)	Increased appetite
	Irritability
	Insomnia
	Swelling in ankles and feet
	Heartburn
	Muscle weakness
	Slow wound healing
	Increased sugar level in blood
	Headache
	Dizziness
	Mood swings
	Cataracts and bone thinning after long-term use
Deltasone (prednisone)	Common but not predictable:
	Nausea
	Vomiting
	Loss of appetite
	Heartburn
	Insomnia

Drug	Potential Side Effects
	Sweating
	Acne
	Less common:
	Muscle pain/cramps
	Irregular heartbeat
	Weakness
	Swelling hands/ankles/feet
	Unusual weight gain
	Signs of infection such as fever or persistent sore throat
	Vision problems (such as blurred vision)
	Severe stomach/abdominal pain
	Mental/mood changes
	Slow wound healing
	Thinning skin
	Bone pain
	Menstrual period changes
	Puffy face
	Seizures
	Easy bruising/bleeding
	Elevated blood sugar
	Serious allergic reactions such as rash, itching/swelling
	Severe dizziness
	Trouble breathing
Elotuzumab (no brand name)	When used in combination with Revlimid and low-dose dexamethasone:
	Low white blood cell counts
	Low platelet counts/low red blood cell counts
	Nausea

Drug	Potential Side Effects
	Dizziness
	Fever
Kyprolis (carfilzomib)	Anemia
	Thrombocytopenia or low platelet count in the blood
	Fatigue
	Nausea
	The FDA has noted:
	Seventy percent of myeloma patients in phase II trials had mild to moderate lung-related side effects such as shortness of breath, blood clots in the lung, and fluid accumulation in the lungs.
	Nine deaths in a clinical trial group of 526 myeloma patients occurred; most if not all were due to heart-related issues that these patients had before beginning the trial.
Pomalyst (pomalidomide)	Suddenly lowered blood pressure, producing dizziness or imbalance upon standing
	Skin rash
	Constipation
	Edema, which is swelling due to excess water retention
	Peripheral neuropathy, mild to moderate tingling or burning sensations and decreased sensitivity in hands or feet
	Anemia-related fatigue, excess bleeding, and infection
	Blood clots
	Severe birth defects or fetal death
Revlimid (lenalidomide)	Blood clots, particularly when taken in combination with steroids or chemotherapy
	Low blood counts; possibly white cell, red cell, platelet, or a combination of them

Drug	Potential Side Effects
	Rash
	Itchy scalp
	Diarrhea
	Fatigue
	Muscle cramps
Thalomid (thalidomide)	Blood clots, particularly when taken in combination with steroids or chemotherapy
	Peripheral neuropathy; numbness or tingling in hands or feet
	Sensations of sedation or fatigue
	Constipation
	Rash, usually on chest, back, arms, legs
	Severe birth defects if taken during pregnancy
Velcade (bortezomib)	Peripheral neuropathy; numbness or tingling in hands or feet
	Low platelet count
	Weakness and fatigue
	Loss of appetite, nausea, vomiting
	Diarrhea or constipation
	Joint pain, muscle cramps
	Shortness of breath, dizziness, blurred vision
	Increased risk of shingles*

* Expect your doctor to consider prescribing acyclovir to protect you from shingles during the time you take Velcade. Acyclovir has no noticeable side effects.

Side Effects in General

	Notes and Measures You Can Take
Anemia (low red blood cell count)	Symptoms are fatigue, listlessness, and pale appearance. Blood tests such as the complete blood count (CBC) will reveal this condition. Your medical team will evaluate its severity and prescribe countermeasures
Constipation	Drink more water
	Drink warm beverages before bowel movements
	Eat foods high in fiber
	Use stool softeners, laxatives, or fiber-binding agents such as Metamucil and Citracil
	Relax and take your time for bowel movements
	Increase physical activity
Diarrhea	Medications that may cause diarrhea include:
	Laxatives
	Antibiotics
	Antacids with magnesium
	Antidepressants
	Some prescription meds. Read the labels.
	Herbal supplements that may cause diarrhea:
	Milk thistle
	Aloe
	Cayenne
	Saw palmetto
	Ginseng
	Coping with diarrhea:
	Increase fluid intake: Water, Ricelyte, Pedialyte, sports drinks such as Gatorade, diluted fruit juice, broth

	Notes and Measures You Can Take
	Avoid caffeinated, carbonated, or heavily sugared beverages
	Fiber-binding agents such as Metamucil or Citracil
	Imodium, Lomotil, or another compound recommended by your doctor
Infection	Stay away from people with infectious disease
	Wash your hands frequently
	Tell your doctor if you feel sick
	Keep your flu shots current
	Get pneumonia vaccine shot
	Get intravenous immune globulin infusions
	Make sure the neutrophil content in your blood is adequate
Nausea	Concentrate on staying hydrated
	Eat before getting very hungry
	Eat bland food—cold or at room temperature
	Find fresh air
	Use relaxation techniques
	Try hypnosis, acupuncture, or acupressure devices such as Sea-Bands
	Restrict fluids with meals
	Chew slowly and thoroughly
	Suck on mints, hard candy, ice pops, or ice chips
	Try peppermint or ginger tea
	Apply a cool compress to the forehead, neck, wrists
	If nausea persists, talk to your doctor about prescription remedies
Neuropathy (numbness or tingling in hands or feet)	Report it to your medical team. Meanwhile:

	Notes and Measures You Can Take
	Massage the area. Cocoa butter helps sometimes
	Take glutamine (vitamin B-complex vitamin supplement)
	Take folic acid (Neurontin)
	Your doctor may prescribe:
	Lidoderm patch or gabapentin
	Physical therapy
	Reduce or stop taking Thalomid, Revlimid, or Velcade
Neutropenia (low white cell count)	Symptoms are fever, shaking, and chills. Sometimes dizziness or fainting. Blood tests such as the CBC will reveal this condition. Your medical team will evaluate its severity and prescribe countermeasures. With a fever over 100.5°, this may require hospitalization to get IV antibiotics
Osteoporosis (bone health)	Your doctor may prescribe:
	Bisphosphonates, such as Actonel, Actonel + Ca, Aredia, Boniva, Didronel, Fosamax, Fosamax + D, Reclast, Skelid, and Zometa to improve bone health.
	Exercise is important to bone health. The National Institutes of Health recommends weight training, walking, hiking, jogging, climbing stairs, tennis, and dancing
Thrombocytopenia (low platelet count)	Symptoms include easy bruising, blood in stool or urine, nosebleeds, cuts that won't stop bleeding. Blood tests such as the CBC will reveal this condition. Your medical team will evaluate its severity and prescribe countermeasures
	Don't take aspirin

	Notes and Measures You Can Take
	Don't take nonsteroidal anti-inflammatory drugs such as Advil, Motrin, Nuprin, Medipren, Aflaxen, Aleve, Anaprox, Midol Extended Relief, Naprelan, Naprosyn, Rx-Act All Day Pain Relief, and Wal-Proxen
	Avoid contact sports and heavy lifting
	Vitamin therapy
	Curcumin or turmeric
	Vitamin B6 protects nerve endings
	Folate helps red cells form
	Herbs and teas are often suggested. Proceed cautiously. For example, Velcade and green tea or Velcade and vitamin C are known to cause toxic reactions
Vomiting	Avoid strong odors
	Don't lie flat after eating
	Avoid sweet, salty, fatty, spicy, citrus, tomatoes, and heavy foods
	Don't exercise after eating
	If you suspect you are going to vomit, eat things you don't particularly like, not favorite foods. Foods that one vomits become things that one will not look forward to eating again
	Nausea medicine also helps stop vomiting

Coming Soon: Chocolate Covered Revlimid

Chemical compounds in chocolate may protect against cancer.

—Melissa Gaskill, "Sweet Relief: Food for Thought," Cure Magazine, Summer 2012

Cocoa, the raw material in chocolate, contains compounds named catechins and proanthocyanidins, members of a class of plant chemicals called flavonols, says Gertraud Maskarinec, MD, PhD, professor at the University of Hawaii Cancer Center. In a recent study published in *Molecular Nutrition & Food Research,* he notes that cocoa blocked cell-signaling pathways involved in tumor formation and seemed to reduce oxidative stress.

In another study at the Lombardi Comprehensive Cancer Center, Georgetown University, proanthocyanidins appeared to deactivate forces that encourage cancer cells to multiply.

These compounds act as antioxidants, says Kathy Allen, a registered dietitian and director of nutrition at the H. Lee Moffitt Cancer Center & Research Institute, Tampa, Florida. Normal breathing produces free radicals, which can cause cell damage and inflammation, both of which are associated with cancer risk. Antioxidants help rid the body of free radicals and help cells repair themselves, possibly reducing the risk of cancer.

Anti-inflammatory and antioxidant foods can potentially protect people from cancer at three stages, says David L. Katz, MD, Director of the Yale-Griffin Prevention Research Center. First, they can lower the rate of mutation. Second, by preventing inflammation or an excess of free radicals, antioxidants give our immune systems the upper hand in destroying abnormal cell lines that can result from mutations. Finally, these nutrients may help prevent those cell lines from becoming malignant.

Exactly what these compounds do in the body is still under investigation, Professor Maskarinec says. They may stimulate immune response, modulate detoxifying enzymes, regulate hormone metabolism, control programmed cell death, or reduce abnormal cell proliferation.

More research is also needed to determine how much cocoa should be consumed for protective benefits without undesirable side effects, such as (horrors!) weight gain.

We know that things we like are sinful. If a food exists that fights cancer, it's going to be okra, not chocolate. But maybe, just this once, some small piece of myeloma's drug scene could be tasty. And maybe—after all the high-priced help in Hawaii, D.C., Florida, and Connecticut has finished scarfing up the lab samples—Hershey, Pennsylvania, will offer concierge services.

12

How to Deal with Chemo: What to Do and How to Do It

You have active roles and responsibilities in an effective chemo program.

Chemotherapy is the systematic treatment of *any* infirmity, using drugs, over a period of time, according to a treatment plan. The daily baby aspirin one takes for heart health is a form of chemotherapy.

The discussion here centers on the sort of chemo that comes as liquids in bags and bottles, that get dripped into patients' veins—often with added ingredients to minimize discomfort and side effects—to fight myeloma.

Your disease is a blood cancer, capable of attack anywhere that blood circulates. Chemo is blood-borne medicine. All myeloma patients receive chemotherapy. All myeloma patients benefit.

"If you've ever had the fortune/misfortune of being injected with this stuff, it won't surprise you to learn

> that it all started with a group of people getting accidentally mustard-gassed in World War I.
>
> When doctors found that the victims developed low white blood cell counts they figured that anything that kills off fast-growing white blood cells might do the same thing to cancers affecting those same cells. Soon other drugs were developed to target the mitosis of cancer cells (were you paying attention in eighth-grade biology?). Drugs that impaired such division are called cytotoxic, naturally, because saying it any other way would make it understandable."
>
> —*John Bogert*
>
> Cancer survivor
>
> *Daily Breeze* newspaper
>
> Torrance, California
>
> May 31, 2011

Wade into the Drug Company's Accompanying Literature

The decision to place you in chemotherapy and the selection of drugs to be used are your doctor's responsibilities. Your job is to remember the names of the drugs, if possible, and most certainly to know what each one is intended to do for you. As you will come to realize, these responsibilities are not trivial.

It is in the nature of those who deal with this complex, critical, and somewhat unpredictable therapy to discuss it using a vocabulary that is foreign and intimidating. With apologies, there are no common words to describe your condition or its treatment; technical jargon is all they got. If they were to depart from the language they learned in school and from one another, all would be lost. Embrace the new lingo and learn what you can.

Should what your medical team is talking about stir your academic juices, put out thirty bucks for a 3 1/2-pound, 988-page wonder titled, *Everyone's Guide to Cancer Therapy, Fifth Edition* by Andrew H. Ko, MD, Malin Dollinger, MD, and Ernest H. Rosenbaum, MD. Some of the smartest men and women on this green earth have labored through five editions and at least a thousand years of clinical practice to bring this explanation of state-of-the-art oncology to the common man.

Your Side of the Street

What may not be explained, and what you will learn here, are matters that you the patient need to know about: what they'll do to you, how to prepare, how you'll feel, and future consequences you might be advised to prepare for.

To reiterate, because there are no more important messages in this book: Keep abreast of what your medical team is thinking and doing. Understand as much as possible. Also keep clear the distinction between patient and doctor. You are the patient. Patients have responsibilities, too, and they are different from those of your medical team.

The Chemo Experience

Unless you are very weak or have medical complications that require it, chemo for myeloma is an outpatient therapy. You go to the chemo room, often called an infusion center or *short stay* if it is in a hospital. You weigh in. Have your temperature taken. If you appear to be fit and free of communicable disease, the nurses help you pick a place to settle in for your treatment and make you comfortable.

Next, your chemo *protocol* will be reviewed and the labels of the medications you will receive will be examined with you. This is a bit like the flight attendant's last check before they close the cabin door: *Everybody's going to Cleveland, right?*

They'll find a vein, probably in your arm or on the back of your hand. They'll stick an IV needle in and tape it down to keep the connection secure. Several small vials of your blood are usually taken for lab analysis.[7] A tube is then attached, running down from bags of fluids hanging above you. A drip, drip, drip begins.

One would think that there would be some sensation from this. The most likely thing is that you'll begin to feel chilly. After a few minutes the recently refrigerated fluids will make you appreciate socks and a warm blanket. You will also be encouraged to drink water. Chemo, surprisingly, can cause dehydration. You may also get sleepy.

The first time you receive chemo, your infusion staff will regulate the flow of medicine to a crawl to keep you from feeling nausea.[8] Later in the session, as your body adjusts, the drip is set faster and faster.

---

7 A complete blood count, as everyone calls it, is a score card by which your medical team grades your progress. A "chemistry panel"—additional blood feature analysis—is also frequently performed. You will learn a lot about your condition by having a doctor or nurse go over these tests results with you. Ask for copies of these reports. Keep a chronological file to look back at later and quite possibly, to answer future questions from medical teams and others with an important need to know.

8 Years ago, nausea during chemo was common and sometimes severe. A NASA astronaut's name will be forever associated with the program that brought you today's effective antinausea meds: ... Jake Garn has made a mark in the Astronaut Corps because he represents the maximum level of space sickness that anyone can ever attain, and so the mark of being totally sick and totally incompetent

Clearly, your treatment team wants the best experience for you. But the fact is that your reaction to chemo drugs can range from mild discomfort to feeling like you've been run over by a truck. If the experience of the chemo room staff is that a particular protocol will be easy on you, your nurse is very apt to volunteer the happy assurance. When they begin your chemo session with Tylenol, Benadryl, and Valium, they are trying to make a difficult time more tolerable.

History and Its Lessons

Chemo earned a bad rep 40 years ago. Latent fear and folklore remain. But that was then. This is now. You will look back on your chemo and say that, while life has held greater joys, it was not that bad.

Right now, as you contemplate the road ahead, you are apt to hear things that worry you. Some of them are true. Some are told in the grand tradition of war story exaggeration. The worst matters are that you may lose your hair, and that you will suffer side effects.

> "My husband's gone with me to all of my chemotherapy sessions. He's my chemosabe."

---

is one Garn. Most guys will get maybe to a tenth Garn, if that high. Interview with Robert E. Stevenson, MD, Johnson Space Center Oral History Project. May 13, 1999, p.35.

—Myeloma support group humor

Take a Spouse or Close Friend to Chemo with You

At least in the beginning, don't go to chemo alone. All sorts of large and small reasons for sharing the experience with a spouse or a good friend will turn up. Among them: After you're hooked up to the tubes and comfy, you may want someone to get you a magazine or a snack. Or you may want to have someone take care of matters in the business office. Or the book you took to pass the time got old and you want someone to talk to.

At least in the beginning, someone should drive you home. Have a suitable waterproof bag handy in case you experience motion sickness, which can come on suddenly.

What to Wear

Wear comfortable casual clothes. Don't wear anything that might be ruined by a spill. Sleeves should be short or easy to push out of the way for blood pressure reading and IV installation.

Since chemo is normally received in a big easy chair or a hospital bed, women may find slacks more comfortable than a skirt. Jewelry and makeup are optional.

Perfume, shaving lotion, or any other thing you wear that has a scent is not good. There are apt to be patients nearby with respiratory complications or heightened sensitivity to odors.

If you can, leave valuables locked in the car or at home. You are apt to nap or go to the bathroom. Why worry about stuff you didn't need to bring?

A physical examination before or after chemo may require that you disrobe. Chemo will not. If an IV entry point has been surgically installed—a port-a-cath or a PICC-line[9]—wear a shirt that allows easy access to it.

Random Thoughts as You Prepare for Chemo

Accept the adventure. Embrace it.

Many physicians and staff pray for their patients. Rarely with them, but privately, for them. There would

---

9 Some patients will be given a surgically implanted entry point for IV in the high chest called a port-a-cath, or a peripherally inserted central catheter (PICC) in the upper arm. Physicians order them for comfort, convenience, and patient safety—most often when the patient's veins are fragile, hard to find, and when the IV fluid is caustic (vesicant).

be benefits should you also speak to the god of your understanding in prayer.

Direct calls to the chemo room are the best way to get information on events and for clarification of things that you did not understand. Your call is also appreciated if you'll be late. The administration of time slots and dose management are helped by your thoughtfulness. Please don't make frivolous calls, and be brief.

Before you go to chemo, finish whatever needs to be done that day. Until you gain some experience, plan nothing after chemo, except maybe a nap.

In that same regard, if children are living with you, consider scheduling a play day for them somewhere else.

Ask family, your boss at work, and others who habitually involve you in stressful matters to cool it. Make it a formal request. Be insistent. Stress relief is a necessary part of the healing process during chemo.

Make your last meal before chemo something light and bland. Don't drink alcohol or take any vitamin, drug, or herb that the oncology team doesn't know about.

There are those who return to a busy schedule after chemo. You may be able to do that, too. If so, it is more apt to happen later in the experience than after the first or second session; your body needs time to develop tolerance to the treatment.

Get someone to take your picture all hooked up. It is a useful way to help others understand what you are going through.

Do's and Don'ts at the Clinic

Chemo becomes a recurring event in the lives of those who must receive it. Learn the names of the staff. Meet other patients. Be friendly. Your stay will be far more pleasant.

Take a note pad. If you don't understand what's going on, ask. If you can't get a satisfactory answer, write a memo so that you will remember to bring it up with the right person later.

Bring a happy book to enjoy, or a DVD you can play (with earphones) on your laptop.

Allow yourself to be pampered.

Staff and patients often stock a table with snacks to be communally shared. Enjoy and participate in this harmless decadence. Eat conservatively to avoid unsettling consequences.

You will notice other patients napping. Feel free to join them.

Please don't plan to spend time on your cell phone, unless you are receiving chemo in a private place. It is oafish to force your phone conversation on others.

If You Are Going to Lose Your Hair

At the time your physician prescribes chemo, hair loss ought to be mentioned if it is possible. If the subject doesn't come up, you are probably safe, but ask anyway. You need to know for sure.

- If you are going to lose your hair, a handout will probably come with the news. It will answer most if not all of your questions.
- Medicare does not reimburse for wigs. Other insurance may, with a prescription from your doctor for a *cranial prosthesis.*
- The American Cancer Society would like to help. For advice and free wigs for cancer patients, and for recommended sales outlets, call 800-850-9445.
- If you decide to buy a wig, get it beforehand so that the fitter and stylist can do their best for you. Cost range is from $40 to $thousands.
- Men: A bad rug looks worse than bald.
- Bald can look very good on some women, too.
- Hats and scarves can be suitable wig substitutes. Cost is less. Comfort is greater. Or get a variety of hats and hair. It'll entertain your grandchildren and stir 'em up at church.
- If you lose your hair, you'll probably lose your eyebrows, too. Eyelash loss is less likely. You will

hear all about these and other details when you start the wig and alternative head cover conversations with people.

- In most cases, hair regrows as soon as the chemo is over.

Pain or Numbness in Hands or Feet: Neuropathy

Everyone with myeloma will experience weird sensations in hands and feet some of the time. It's a side effect of your condition and can get worse or occur more often after you start chemo. Be careful when you experience it. You can hurt yourself and not realize it. Or you may not realize how serious the injury is.

The Fog That Follows Chemo—Chemo Brain

Don't be surprised if your ability to concentrate is lessened by chemotherapy or if you have some short-term memory loss. Problems with word retrieval, processing numbers, following instructions, multitasking, and setting priorities are common. Symptoms are most apparent in individuals who are used to juggling the demands of complex lives.

Most patients get their clear heads back shortly after completing chemo, but about 15% suffer a prolonged effect of what is medically known as *chemotherapy-induced cognitive impairment.*

Several recently published books on this phenomenon are considered authoritative and helpful. Reviewers rate *Your Brain After Chemo* (Da Capo Press, 2010), by Daniel H. Silverman, MD, and Idelle Davidson, as most user friendly.

Chemo May Open the Door to Infection and Reduced Vitality

Your chemo will destroy bone marrow, the birthplace of fresh blood cells along with malignant myeloma cells. The trick is to balance the ingredients in the chemo cocktail so that it kills more of the bad guys than the good.

What your doc wants to avoid is the destruction of too many red blood cells, causing anemia (fatigue and loss of energy); or damage to platelets, causing thrombocytopenia (bruising, nose and gum bleeds); or loss of white cells, causing neutropenia (which makes you more susceptible to infection).

Neutropenia—very low white cell count—is the worst and most dangerous of the three. Fatigue, body aches, swelling, and redness are usual symptoms. Sometimes a low-grade fever is the only sign. A temp of 100.5° can herald a condition called *febrile neutropenia,* which requires immediate hospitalization.

The Effects of Your Chemo Will Vary

A myeloma patient presents a puzzle to medical science that is complex beyond belief. Your blood, bones, and affected organs have constantly changing features that will determine which chemotherapy drugs work best for you. It is very important that you be in the hands of a sophisticated treatment team that pays attention to every nuance.

As an example, during the progress of your disease one of the chromosomes in IgH, a constituent of your blood, may become displaced. When that happens, the chemo you had been receiving may become less effective, or begin producing new, unwanted side effects. Current thinking among scientists is that somewhere between 20% and 60% of myeloma patients get this condition.

Don't be overly concerned about it. There are countermeasures. It's just another one of those unexpected blows that can come along during treatment. Sometimes winning doesn't feel like it.

Your chemotherapy should effectively thwart your myeloma. It will give you a better shot at a longer, higher-quality life, with fewer side effects, than patients enjoyed even a few years ago.

> Chemotherapy is part science, part art, with no guarantee and no warranty period.

Health Tips

Chemotherapy often compromises the immune system's ability to fight off viral invaders. Your degree of susceptibility and the length of time before your system's natural defenses come back are not predictable, though most *healthy* people—just myeloma, no other major complaints—sail through this.

So:

- If you are preparing for a transplant procedure or just coming home after one, you will want to observe all these tips.
- If your chemo has another purpose, this much precaution would be a bit over the top.

Ask your doc for guidance.

Recommendation	Comment
Don't put off or interrupt your chemo.	You have a progressive disease.
	Don't give it further free rein.
Wash your hands after exposure to germs or infection.	Use warm water and soap. Scrub for at least 20 seconds. Waterless antibacterial lotion also works.
Use air purifiers at home and work.	For the best product, explain your need to the supplier and get a recommendation.

Recommendation	Comment
Aspirin may not be an ideal pain reliever for you.	Some over-the-counter pain relievers may not be suitable during chemo. Ask your doctor for a recommendation.
Insist on clean, healthy friends.	Ask visitors to have clean hands and not to bring communicable diseases near you. Gowns and face masks are excessive precautions.
No manicures, pedicures, or other procedures that cut or abrade your skin.	Exceptionally serious infection can result.
Get dental work, including cleaning, done before starting chemo.	Consult with your oncologist before any dental procedure during chemo.
Avoid crowded public places.	Gathering places such as worship centers, stadiums, and public transit vehicles are ripe with infection. Teachers should consider sabbaticals. When crowding is unavoidable, wear a facemask.
Play only with healthy children.	No diaper changing. No wiping noses. Don't touch excrement or vomit.
Reduce stress.	Stay away from angry people. Keep work hours short.
Avoid travel.	Best to stay home. Travel to a third-world country would be insane.
Start chemo with up-to-date inoculations.	Flu, tetanus, pneumonia, and any other precautionary inoculation your oncologist recommends should be completed before starting chemo.
Stay out of the sun.	Your skin may become extra sensitive during chemo. Sunburn can be nasty.
If you garden...	Don't.

Recommendation	Comment
Learn and practice sterile procedures in the kitchen.	Keep dishes and work surfaces very clean. Empty trash promptly. Keep the garbage disposal clear. Clean the refrigerator. No bugs, especially winged ones.
Be careful of raw fruits and vegetables.	Have someone else, whose sanitary practices you trust, wash and peel it for you. Eat immediately.
No uncooked seafood	Not even sushi or freshly shucked oysters.
Don't eat alfalfa sprouts.	This is an ingeniously eclectic plant.
Don't eat raw dairy.	Raw milk is hard to find, but raw cheese is a featured item in many deli counters.
Slice foods at home.	Don't buy sliced deli meats. Thoroughly clean and cook products from the butcher's case.
Wear gloves when performing any cleaning chore.	If a glove tears, remove it, wash the hand, then put on a new glove before resuming.
Use a hand can opener.	Wash after use.
Defrost foods in the refrigerator or microwave.	Never thaw on the counter.
Set the refrigerator temperature at 40°F or less. Set the freezer at 0°F.	Some foods may be unintentionally ruined by the excess cold. Consider those to be acceptable losses.
Pets are a health problem.	No animal is clean enough for you to kiss or snuggle. Don't clean up urine or feces. Don't change the birdcage liner. Don't let your dog lick you.
Keep your teeth clean.	Use a soft-bristled brush and nonabrasive cleaner.

Recommendation	Comment
Don't vacuum.*	Wait for three months after chemo before entering a room in which a vacuum is operating, or was, in the last hour or two.

[* Cleaning for a Reason will have a participating maid service in your zip code clean your home once a month for four months while you are undergoing chemo, no charge. Sign up at www.cleaningforareason.org. Get your doctor to fax the company an attesting note.]

Don't Hide Unless You Have To

You don't have to avoid friends and family unless your doctor tells you that you should. Even though myeloma and its treatments have compromised your immune system, you may still be able to enjoy those you love. Ask your doctor what precautions you should take.

Professionals Who Need to Know About Your Chemo

Dentists, pharmacists, ophthalmologists, nutritionists, purveyors of Chinese medicine, chiropractors, and others who support your good health—all need to know about your disease and treatment. So does a case nurse at your health maintenance organization or preferred provider organization. Any of them may have helpful insights for you.

In this complex, very serious circumstance, there needs to be a chief executive. You have very wisely given that role to your oncologist. When suggestions or recommendations come to you from others, you help everybody by airing the subject with your team's CEO.

Your Dentist

Chemo can cause gum disease and tooth decay. Have a copy of your oncologist's treatment protocol sent to your dentist. Then consult. Your dentist may need to examine you during or following chemo, or may prescribe a special regimen of oral hygiene.

Your Ophthalmologist

Another copy of your treatment protocol should go to your eye doctor. Cataracts and other eye disease may be side effects of chemo. The American Ophthalmological Society advises even people with 20/20 vision and seemingly perfect eye health to be checked after chemo.

To clarify a point of common misunderstanding, the eye doctor we are discussing holds an MD degree and perhaps a secondary oncology credential. When selecting a medical professional to serve this important need, look for the MD after the person's name. There are others in related specialties—who may also be called *doctor*—who are not qualified to serve you in this circumstance.[10]

Your Pharmacist

You now rely on the ministrations of multiple medical specialties, any of whom may prescribe for you. Some of them shortcut the prescription process and just hand you something. Though they all endorse the logic of controlled substance management, they don't share information. You are the only one who speaks to them all.

Pick a pharmacist who will agree to list and track all the drug prescriptions you get from all the places you go for treatments. Keep this person advised of everything you take, including herbs and other health food products. Expect to receive invaluable commentary and alerts to drug interactions that should then go to the oncologist leading your health care team.

---

10 The competence of the individual is not the only matter. Your insurance may not cover the treatment if provided by anyone other than an MD.

Your Health Insurance and Medicare/Medicaid

Your health care plan administrators' rule book is not generous in its allowances for dentistry, eye disease, chiropractic, Chinese medicine, acupuncture, and nutritional consultation during chemo. Be prepared for an automatic rejection when you open the subject of coverage. *This* would be a *very* good time to start the slog through the clearance processes. Call your Medicare/Medicaid and insurance company's claim numbers *right now.* Your oncologist may also have to weigh in personally so that health insurance managers understand how these chemo-induced needs differ from the usual, customarily discounted health services.

13

Rules for Radiation: Huge Machinery Simply Explained

A ray of hope from the Plains of Barsoom. [11]

The Ray Gun Comes to Life

Marie Skłodowska-Curie was first to experiment with radiation as a treatment for cancer. Hers was a towering intellect, fighting for acceptance in the 1890s; at a time when science was men-only; further handicapped by being young, and attractive, and in Paris.

One hopes she appreciated the irony, when a bunch of penny-a-line romance novelists, led by H.G. Wells, began arming pulp fiction characters with ray guns and clouding their worlds with mysterious radioactive gases. Imagine the only female professor of the Sorbonne as *War of the Worlds, A Princess of Mars,* and Amazing Stories comic books trivialized the science that had made her a Nobel laureate.

---

11 The setting of A Princess of Mars, Edgar Rice Burroughs, 1916.

So began the world's fascination with radiation—waves of energy. While people are still trying to invent Buck Rogers's blaster, the guns in medicine, aimed at myeloma, are ready.

The First Rule for Radiation

Avoid unnecessary x-rays, computed tomography (CT), and positron emission tomography (PET) scans. Radiation builds up in the body. The eventual cumulative dose can cause disease. Professor Curie died in 1934 of aplastic anemia, brought about by her research.

Codicil to the First Rule

Don't refuse the radiation that your myeloma treatment team wants for you. They know what they're doing and will keep you safe.

However ... you are an interesting subject. You have a rare cancer. Other physicians and researchers in the oncology community may want to know how you are progressing in your fight against myeloma and to examine you to learn more about why. It is advisable for you to consult with your medical team before accepting offers to participate in optional studies that require x-ray, CT, or PET examinations.

Clarification of the Codicil

To avoid confusing closely related subjects, rely on two key nouns: radiation *therapy* and radiation *imaging.*

Radiation *therapy* is a huge subject. We are only going to cover the part of it that destroys myeloma cells and relieves certain other conditions you may face. The specialty that uses this science for your benefit, called *radiation oncology,* is a branch of care performed by a medical doctor.

X-rays and other *imaging* use the same science, but just for reconnaissance. This is a general diagnostic technique that many specialties in medicine—doctors, dentists, chiropractors—rely on. A physician qualified to interpret x-ray imaging is a radiologist.

More Hope Than Promise

Radiation oncology is a work in progress. Some gray-haired guy, with titles and honors and degrees up one arm and down the other, may tell you that the result of a radiological procedure you have gone through is unclear. Or that you need to keep coming back for more of the same, even though everyone is pretty sure they've destroyed the cancer site. That sort of ambiguity is part of the nature of this thing. You can feel confident that you have benefited from the state of the art. Despite the impressive size and complexity of the equipment, it is art, however, not certainty.

As with other matters on the myeloma journey, you will benefit by assuring yourself that the radiation treatments you receive are the latest and best, in the hands of outstanding men and women of science. You do that by keeping your treatment conversation ongoing and by listening to those on your treatment team discuss your status and options. When you hear confidence, feel assured. If somebody says to you, *Well, this is as good as you can get unless...,* find out more about going to the place, or doing the thing, that the *unless* refers to.

The Arsenal

During your treatment trip down myeloma lane, you are going to be served by radiation in three ways: imaging devices that are general information gatherers; imaging devices that guide surgeons and radiation oncologists during procedures; and radiation as a tool that damages cancer cells so they die.

Imaging Devices Used for Information or as Guides for Procedures

The tendency with radiation equipment is to make each successive model bigger, better, and more expensive. It's the American way. It may also lead you to believe that your session will feature a type of equipment not on the generic list that follows. Not so. One of this list's terms will be found somewhere in the name on the device or on the door of the lab you enter to use it.

CT	Computed tomography (CT) shows an area's cross section. Often many cross sections are made at regular intervals. When they are laid out, shapes can be seen in three dimensions.
	The process is the same as if you put a hard-boiled egg through a slicer. You could look at the slices one by one to see the shape that the yolk had within the white, very exactly.
MRI	In magnetic resonance imaging (MRI), a large, powerful magnet causes cell nuclei to produce magnetic fields detectable by the scanner. Some are stronger than others, allowing the equipment to create very detailed two- or three-dimensional pictures.
	An MRI can spot soft tumors in bone marrow, and make similarly fine distinctions between other soft tissues. It is uniquely valuable for some studies of your disease.
	The strong magnetic fields used for MRI are harmless, though you must leave metal objects such as belt buckles in the dressing room, along with credit cards and gadgets with erasable data.
PET	A positron emission tomography (PET) scan uses a radioactive substance called a tracer to look for disease in the body. It lights up the area of interest when the scanner looks at it.
	The isotope becomes harmless after a short time and leaves in the urine.
	You are close enough to being nonradioactive to leave isolation after the procedure. You may, however, still setoff a security magnetometer for a day or two. If you must fly or visit a building with heightened security, such as a big city mayor's office, bring documentation to explain why the alarm bells are sounding.

Ultrasound	This is imaging using sound wave echoes. The view is not quite as good as an x-ray but very safe.
X-ray	X-band energy is sent through you. The area of interest casts a shadow onto a piece of film, a sensitized plate, or is captured like a TV signal and displayed on a screen.

They Don't Take Color Pictures

Imaging always starts in a digital form—zeros and ones—black and white. So digital imaging must start as *mono* (one) *chrome* (color). When it is helpful, these groupings of zeros and ones can be assigned colors by a computer. Any color pictures you're shown of scenes from inside your body were constructed in this way.

Radiation Therapy, the Sharp End of the Stick

Radiation therapy has been used to treat cancer for 100 years. Today, about 70% of myeloma patients with bone lesions will benefit from it. Other conditions caused by myeloma also invite the ray gun. Taken together, you can be fairly certain that radiation oncology will benefit you sometime in the not-too-distant future.

Specialty Treatment Programs

Helical Tomotherapy

The TomoTherapy® HI-ART® Treatment System, manufactured by Accuracy, Inc., represents the latest generation of technology, delivering radiation therapy with surgical precision, according to experts. This means more effective treatment, with reduced damage to nearby healthy tissue and organs.

Older methods of radiation therapy focus larger beams of radiation from two to six different directions. This system uses hundreds of thinner beams, spirally rotating around the tumor, focusing in from all directions.

Previous treatments required two separate apparatuses—one to view the target, one to deliver radiation. With helical tomotherapy, a CT scanner is married to the radiation source. The CT locks onto the treatment site, like a jet fighter's radar locks onto an enemy plane. As the patient lies on a treatment couch with the tomotherapy system spiraling, its radiation beam turns on and off rapidly, delivering hundreds of precise hits to the tumor.

Image-Guided Radiation Therapy

Each time you return for treatment you sit or lie in a slightly different position. Even if you could be repositioned exactly, your body parts and tumors would be in slightly different places. Imageguided radiation therapy (IGRT) provides radiation oncologists with the tools to see the tumor better, track its movement, and stay on target. You may hear it said that tomotherapy, which is less apt to damage areas near the malignancy, has replaced standard IGRT at many of today's advanced treatment centers. Probably not true. Tomotherapy is the new kid on the block, but IGRT is most likely still there, still effective, easier, and cheaper if its capabilities are sufficient for your need.

Three-Dimensional Conformal Therapy

Three-dimensional treatment planning uses CT or MRI data to calculate tumor volume and measure the proximity of nearby normal structures. A precisely shaped high dose of radiation can then be delivered to the tumor, while avoiding collateral damage.

Total Body Irradiation

Some stem cell transplant centers combine total body irradiation with high-dose chemotherapy to most effectively kill the patient's myeloma-infested bone marrow, in preparation for transplant. The combo is used when the transplant team believes it will help the patient recover more quickly and in greater comfort.[12]

Brachytherapy

This method of radiation treatment uses sealed radioactive sources placed inside the body at short distances from the patient's tumor. This allows delivery of a higher radiation dose, more precisely, than would be possible with external beam radiation.

Men are most apt to have heard of this technique because it is common in the treatment of prostate cancers.

Radiosurgery

The CyberKnife® System, also manufactured by Accuracy, Inc., is a highly advanced form of robotic radiosurgery. It is a painless noninvasive treatment that delivers high doses of precisely targeted radiation to tumors or lesions. Its flexible robotic arm makes it possible to treat areas such as the spine and spinal cord. (There is no real knife; the product delivers knife-like precision.)

Treatments are performed on an outpatient basis, with each session lasting 30 to 90 minutes. The number of treatments varies depending on the tumor size,

---

12 See Chapter 15, Your Stem Cell Transplant: Lots of Patients Do It, Step Three—Mobilization.

location, and shape. Two to five trips to the *knife* are usually required.

Some conditions may be treated with a different noninvasive radiotherapy device called the gamma knife, which also delivers a single, finely focused, high dose of radiation. The gamma knife is used primarily to treat small benign or malignant brain tumors, epilepsy, trigeminal neuralgia, or abnormal blood vessel formations located in the brain.

Recovery after use of either radio surgical tool is often immediate.

Side Effects from Radiation Therapy

Different people have different side effects after radiation. You may have little or only mild reaction. Someone else may have many or severe side effects. Your radiation oncologist, or a nurse on staff, is apt to have a pretty good idea of how you will do, *if you ask.* Unfortunately, it's impossible to know with certainty. The specific side effects you may have depend on the type of radiation being used, the dose of radiation, the area of the body that's being targeted, and the state of your health.

Some side effects from radiation therapy happen right away, such as skin irritation, hair loss at the radiation site, nausea, or fatigue. Loss of energy may last from hours to several weeks after treatment ends; worse in the beginning, less severe after later treatments.

There are some late side effects, including lung or heart problems that may take years to develop and may not be reversible. That is why special care is taken before radiation near heart or lungs.

What Can I Do About Fatigue?

If radiation therapy leaves you drained of energy, discuss it with your doctor. You'll face a struggle. Time will be your most important healer.

Work with a counselor or take a class offered at your cancer treatment center to learn ways to conserve energy, reduce stress, and use distraction to reduce fatigue. Prioritize your regular activities so you can get most done before you run out of gas.

Maintain a balance between rest and activities. Too much bed rest can make you more fatigued.

Talk with your family and friends and ask for their help. If fatigue is interfering with your job, discuss your situation with your employer and ask about taking some time off from work or making adjustments in your schedule. Keep in mind that the fatigue related to radiation therapy will most likely be temporary and will pass several weeks after your radiation treatment ends.

14

Notes on Surgery: Surgery Plays Supporting Roles

Surgery is important for damage control and pain relief.

Surgery, so often associated with curing cancer, plays support roles in myeloma cases. Surgery frequently improves quality of life and patient comfort. It may stop a threatening condition from becoming worse. But surgery won't cure myeloma.

Sorts of Surgery Ahead

All myeloma patients will need to undergo minor surgical procedures from time to time. The most common of these procedures will most likely be bone marrow biopsies. This relatively simple procedure is often done using only local anesthesia. Some patients experience little discomfort, but for others, the pain can be excruciating, according to Pat Killingsworth, a myeloma patient speaking from too much experience. There are two ways to help ensure a less traumatic experience, he adds. One is to undergo a sedated biopsy. This option is often available at larger cancer centers. Larger centers also use a mechanical driver to take core samples. This lessens postprocedure pain and helps speed recovery. If only local anesthesia is available where you are, ask your doctor to use one of these mechanical drivers instead of a manual coring tool.

Another form of minor surgery common to myeloma patients is catheter implantation, which allows medical staff to start IVs and take blood draws without needing to stick you each time. Catheters may be placed in your arm, chest, or neck. Your doctor will select the type and location that works best for what he or she has planned.

The next most likely forms of surgery are procedures for removal of bone lesions, though most lesions are fixed using radiation; and for making orthopedic repairs, most often in the spine, pelvis, hip, shoulder, or jaw. Bone fractures and bone deformities can be corrected by bone grafting and other bone surgeries. The objectives of these surgeries are to decrease pain and to preserve physical abilities.

You may need an orthopedic surgeon to repair badly weakened bone; to make joint replacement; or to provide what is called *internal fixation augmentation* to supplant a failed structure—notably in your backbone—with cement or splint. If myeloma has advanced before being discovered, these procedures are more likely. When myeloma is caught early, chemo and radiation have a good chance to keep you out of this kind of trouble.

Surgery of a Much Higher, More Complex Nature Is Needed in Some Cases

Untreated myeloma destroys skeletal structure. Excess calcium is released in the bloodstream, which damages vital organs including the liver, the kidneys, and the stomach. Major surgery must follow.

Liver

If your liver is badly damaged, a liver transplant is necessary. This involves grafting a portion or the complete liver from a donor to the patient. Fortunately, liver failure is rare.

Kidney

Kidney damage is common due to the excess calcium in the blood. Your immune system, which should be helping your kidneys, is overtaxed. Surgery, up to and including transplant, may be necessary.

Stomach

Stomach repair is always difficult. The only general comments to be made here are to listen very carefully to what your surgeon has to say and then get a second opinion. Pay particular attention to the outcomes being forecast.

Skeletal Complications

Myeloma-associated bone lesions typically do not heal, even in patients who have been in remission for years. Skeletal complications may, over time, create permanent disabilities, require surgical intervention, and even affect survival. According to a recent study by James Berenson, MD, of the Institute for Myeloma and Bone Cancer Research, a badly compromised skeletal structure leads to a 44% increased likelihood of impending death in myeloma patients. Since the introduction of bisphosphonate treatment[13] for bone disease, the number of myeloma patients requiring surgical intervention for skeletal complications has dropped below 10%. Dr. Berenson adds, "Most commonly performed procedures are minimally invasive procedures for vertebral compression fractures including kyphoplasty or vertebroplasty, procedures for femoral [hip] or humeral [upper arm] fractures including rod placement. Patients who undergo these procedures have a marked improvement in their pain (relief) and mobility."

---

13 Bisphosphonates are also known to cause the death of jawbone tissue by inhibiting the development of blood vessels in the bone, a condition known as osteonecrosis. Ask your oncologist how this may factor in your case. Also see Chapter 11 for more on drugs.

Other Surgery

Middle-aged and older patients often bring other health issues with them to myeloma treatment. Heart disease, stroke, or any of many other major health conditions—including one or more additional forms of cancer—will make myeloma treatment more precarious. Major surgery for one or more of these other afflictions, in the middle of myeloma treatment, can become necessary.

15

Your Stem Cell Transplant: Lots of Patients Do It

A stem cell transplant is equal parts burden and miracle.

Most everybody who has served in the armed forces has some tale to tell about basic training. If you didn't serve, you listen to the talk about crawling through mud while some foul-mouthed sergeant yelled at everybody and you wonder why the spinner of the yarn is smiling about it.

A stem cell transplant is a similar sort of thing for myeloma patients. It's what you do at a point in the myeloma experience to get your life back. There's nothing about it that you will enjoy at the time. But the stories you tell later will bring knowing glances and smiles from all the other vets.

You're in the Army now. No way out of this chicken outfit.

A Stem Cell

There are stem cells in your bone marrow and blood, general-purpose spares that can change into the type of cell that the body needs to repair damage, or in the case that is of most interest here, to establish healthy, myeloma-free bone marrow. Babies have lots of them. By the time we reach adulthood, we have far fewer. They are scarce in seniors but still there.

Bone Marrow Transplant Versus Stem Cell Transplant

Stem cells for transplant were originally taken from the marrow of bones. Now they are usually taken from circulating blood. It's simpler and much easier on the donor.

The circulating blood collection process begins with an injection of a *growth factor,* which helps the body produce a greater number of stem cells. As an important second benefit, the stem cells that are collected in this way have the growth factor within them. So when they are transplanted, they begin to multiply more quickly and into greater volumes of healthy bone marrow.

The Theory

The idea is to wipe out your diseased bone marrow and replace it with healthy new cells. The wiping-out part kills trillions of cells. The replacement step puts back three or four *millionths* of what was taken away. If all things work as expected, the new settlers multiply very rapidly, establishing healthy, myeloma-free bone marrow throughout your body. Bone marrow produces more than 20 billion new blood cells every day throughout a person's life.

Results

In theory, your myeloma is gone. For reasons no one understands, it comes back. For the average person, a transplant keeps the disease away for 2 or 3 years. For some the time is less. For a growing number, 5 or 10 years have passed myeloma free.

Because current treatment technology is only a few years old, *5 or 10 years* is all the history we have to work with. No one knows how long a transplant patient may enjoy recovery.

In about 10% of cases, the implanted stem cell colony does not establish itself and prosper. Should that happen to you, there is a Plan B. Whereas transplant failure presented a bleak picture just a few years ago, myeloma oncology has more effective treatment procedures for *refractory* patients now. Later in this chapter, you will meet Mark Famularo and hear a bit of his story.

> "I think we are all very gratified and excited about the ever prolonged life expectancies in multiple myeloma patients, the SEER data (Annual Surveillance Epidemiology and End Results Report of the National Cancer Institute) that was published this spring showing marked

improvements in survival of multiple myelomas since 1996. It has been very impressive and I think confirms what we have already perceived in our practices ... that change in survival in myeloma essentially corresponds to the year in which transplantation became very preeminent in the Western world as part of the treatment management of multiple myeloma."

—Ann F. Mohrbacher, MD

Oversees myeloma treatment programs at Keck School of Medicine, USC

Those Who Are Eligible Can Expect to Be Told to Get a Transplant

The nation's leading myeloma treatment centers and many physicians of great renown have justified—nevertheless conditioned—opinions. But, assuming you qualify, your doctor is going to recommend that you begin the path toward a stem cell transplant at some point in your treatment. More likely sooner than later.

A transplant ... if you qualify

Not all myeloma patients are candidates for transplant. Not all qualified patients stay eligible.

If you don't know your status, ask your myeloma doctor. If you're eligible, ask your doctor about the things you should do to at least keep all your options open.

In general, the qualifications are:

- Healthy, compatible stem cells must be available.
- Your lung, liver, kidney, and heart status must be good.
- Blood tests must show that the transplant could work.
- The transplant team must believe that you can endure the stress of the procedure.

Compatibility

We, like snowflakes, are all different. But we can have common characteristics. Some of these similarities are necessary for one person to donate new stem cells to another. Same blood type and some genetic compatibility are the driving factors.

Instead of searching for a donor, it's far easier to have your own stem cells *harvested,* to save them while your body is being prepared for transplant, and then have them returned to you. That is called an *autologous* transplant and is a very common, very successful way to go ... if you qualify.

Unlike snowflakes, a few of us are identical twins. If you are in that category, you already know that you can trade blood or cells or even some body parts. A *syngeneic* transplant is the infusion of bone marrow or stem cells from one identical twin into another. And as an identical twin with myeloma you are rare and probably named Kathy Giusti. (Kathy Giusti received stem cells from her identical twin, Karen Andrews, on January 26, 2006. Giusti, diagnosed with the disease in 1998, is founder and chief executive officer, Multiple Myeloma Research Foundation.)

The rest of us have to find a donor. The chance of a brother or sister being a good match is about 1 in 15. The odds of parents or children or anyone else in the family qualifying are 1 in 20,000 or higher; the same odds as matching with the next person you pass on the street. Until recently this could be an insurmountable problem. Now there are large databases of potential donors and computers that make close matching nearly instant. From *close* to *donor-qualified* requires some further sorting and matching.

A transplant using another person's donated cells is called *allogeneic.**

[* Be The Match, operated by the Minneapolis-based National Marrow Donor Program, has more than 8 million potential donors registered. Call 626-256-4673 or go to www.bethematchfoundation.org]

Sometimes patients receive both autologous and allogeneic transplants. Or mini-allogeneic. This has produced the same confusion that 31 flavors created when it added the 32nd carton of ice cream to the freezer. We didn't know we needed Tutti Frutti. Now we can't live without it. God bless science.

Start of the Transplant Journey: Diagnosis, Discussion, Decision

The first thing that happens after a positive myeloma diagnosis is that your case must be evaluated. The next thing is that, from among the treatment options, the conclusion must be reached that a transplant is the best next treatment goal for you. Then you need an independent second opinion that agrees.

In many cases, all this happens automatically. If so, you are on an orderly path. If you don't have a qualified, independent second opinion that agrees with the first one, get one soon. You need to take this step for a dozen reasons—from being sure that you really do have multiple myeloma, to establishing the form and stage of the disease, to the need to file these findings with your health insurance provider to stay in its good graces and to receive maximum support.

Myeloma is a clever, unpredictable, implacable foe. Medics are inclined to go with the process that has brought their patients the greatest levels of success in the past, strongly influenced by:

- The sort of myeloma you have
- Your stamina
- How you feel in general
- Other diseases—such as a heart condition or diabetes—you may have
- The medications you have taken in the past and any changes in your body they may have caused

Your health insurance provider is a central player in all this. *The insurance company* (directly or indirectly) *picks the patient's transplant center, and requires an attending staff led by physicians who specialize in transplant procedures,* says Malin Dollinger, MD, Clinical Professor of Medicine, Keck School of Medicine, USC. A stem cell transplant can easily cost a quarter million dollars. Not to imply that anyone will drag their feet before spending the money. It is more that a transplant is a very big piece on the chessboard and should only be moved after due, deliberate consideration from all points of view.

Study, decide, move. Money you can waste. Time—no.

Mark and Tammy Famularo's Story

At the time of his diagnosis Mark and Tammy had been married nine years. They met at Verizon

Communications where Mark, who had been a lineman for 20 years, was a supervisor and Tammy was an engineer. It had been a second marriage for them, and for the two children each brought to the union. Mark was 44 when he learned of his myeloma.

Mark: *It was June 2004: I needed a work physical. Tests showed blood in my urine so I was referred to a urologist. They thought maybe I had a tear in my bladder. Also I was feeling tired from time to time. Nothing to make me feel that anything was wrong, though.*

In December, I was sent to Dr. Alex Makalinao of California Hematology Oncology Medical Group. The urologist never said it but Dr. Mak did, "By looking at some of these results, there could be cancer but I don't know. Let me do my own tests."

Tammy: *Mark didn't know what an oncologist was. I did because I have a sister who works in oncology as a nurse. But, anyway, we went through a six-month period of testing from June ... They found the M protein in his blood so they did a bone marrow biopsy.*

Mark: *(The evening of the bone marrow biopsy, December 21, 2004) ... Dr. Makalinao was going on vacation and he called me on the phone. He apologized for not seeing me because he was leaving immediately. He said I had bone marrow cancer; multiple myeloma. He wanted me to start chemo right away.*

He wanted to be aggressive with it. Even at that time, he was talking about getting us ready for a transplant.

Tammy: *I got on the Internet and it said ... you've got about three years. Not much information about what to do ... So we were really scared. We had no answers.*

I called my sister, an oncology nurse who works for Dr. Robert Vescio, the director of the Myeloma Program at Cedars-Sinai Medical Center. She spoke to him. He invited us to come in right away because our oncologist wasn't going to be back for a couple of weeks.

Our insurance didn't cover Dr. Vescio so he waived his fee. We saw him within a couple of days. He sat down with us. I had a whole list of questions. He basically went through the disease. What was known about it. What wasn't.

Nothing to suggest how he got it. No link between the toxic materials he was exposed to as a lineman for Verizon and his cancer. It's not genetic ... Mark's always been healthy. Never smoked ... luck of the draw.

The Treatment Plan Is Set

Dr. Mak initiated a chemo-based plan using anti-angiogenesis[14] drugs. The aim was to stabilize Mark's condition, in preparation for stem cell harvest from Mark's blood—a removal process called apheresis[15]—followed by transplant. Mark's key chemo drugs were:

Vincristine
Doxorubicin
Dexamethasone
Cyclophosphamide
Cytoxan

The Reasoning Behind This Chemo Strategy

The body's normal and essential process of encouraging wound healing and cell formation also encourages development of multiple myelomas.

---

14 Named after Genesis, the book in the Bible about creation. These drugs stop the body's cell renewal process. Also called immunomodulators or IMiDs. See Chapter 11, Humuhumunukunukuapuaa: Things to Know About Your Drugs.

15 Apheresis is a procedure that involves drawing blood, separating it into elements that may be removed or treated, and then returning the blood to the patient.

Anti-angiogenesis drugs—drugs that stop cell formation from beginning—are often the first line of attack against freshly discovered myeloma.

Anti-angiogenesis drugs also strangle good cells and stop things that promote health and the person's sense of wellness. Medical science has to be combined with the directing physician's knowledge and instinct as to when to vary the program to ensure that it produces the necessary result with the least possible discomfort and damage to the patient. At the time of Mark's first stem cell transplant in 2005, this process was much more difficult to tolerate than it is today.

Vital Support

Tammy: *We had a transplant coordinator at the UCLA Medical Center: Laura Block, RN, OCN. She was great. Took care of everything ... UCLA, our transplant hospital, is such a maze. I would have been lost without her. She kept us organized and scheduled. All we had to do was show up.*

Mark: *Our first meeting, she walked us through the apheresis and everything that happened after that.*

Tammy: *She scheduled all his labs; the chemo from the very beginning; everything. Very thorough.*

Mark: *Mentally, you're looking at it (thinking) I'm going to do the best I can. You just go with what's ahead ... I don't think stem cell transplant was ever optional for us. I think even now, as we're getting ready to go through a third and fourth one, it's not a choice.*

Tammy: *I was relieved we had any options.*

Mark: *Yeah! As a matter of fact, yeah!*

Tammy: *I remember my Uncle Rodney died of multiple myeloma when I was a kid. It just seemed like they couldn't do much and he died very quickly. So I was very relieved that they could do something for Mark.*

Pretransplant Testing

The chemo process began in January and continued for six months, to the time of Mark's transplant. Key tests, interspersed with chemo infusions, included:

April 27—Nuclear bone scan and chest x-ray
April 28—Echocardiogram
May 2—Pulmonary function, EKG, and blood labs

The Case Nurse

Verizon's group health insurance provider, HealthCare Partners, assigned Jo Taravella, RN, to Mark in January, as a care coordinator, or case nurse. She brought a detailed understanding of resources available through the insurance company to Mark and Tammy, and helped with paperwork.

If you, dear reader, do not know who the Jo Taravella is at your insurance company—your case nurse—call the company, your HMO, or Medicare, or whoever is your primary insurance provider and ask. If you have never spoken to this person, make contact. You need an active, energetic pro who will make things happen in a timely manner, on your behalf, at your insurance company.

The First Transplant, June 2005

Mark: *Day one is getting checked in. Getting relaxed. Getting used to this room, maybe 10 x 15. You've got a TV. Tammy bought me an iPod. You know you're going to be there for at least two weeks, depending on how you [respond to the transplant procedure].*

Day two, they're getting you ready.

Day three, they start the melphalan; the myeloma killer. It's powerful stuff. The next few days were very uncomfortable.*

[* Melphalan (trade name Alkeran) is a chemotherapy drug belonging to the class of alkylating agents. It is used primarily to treat multiple myeloma and ovarian cancer, and occasionally malignant melanoma. Otherwise known as l-phenylalanine mustard, or L-PAM, melphalan is a phenylalanine derivative of mechlorethamine, also called nitrogen mustard. The agent was first used to combat melanoma. It did not work but was found to be of use in myeloma. www.myelomabeacon.com]

What I would tell somebody who will go through this is, look, be ready for two, maybe two and a half weeks, of ups and downs. When I walked in I felt good. Later, I could hardly get up. I needed Tam for everything ... Then I gradually got better and soon I was thinking, man I want out of here.

The worst part of the first week was that I had bad sores at the base of my tongue. When I would talk, they would rub my teeth. And I'm locked in this room with the blower (air sanitizer) going. That first (transplant), I did very little walking in the hallways. I couldn't wait to get home and into that easy chair by the window and feel the breeze. (Because) ... you're so confined. And you miss everybody.

Once you're home, you're around family, your outlook's different. For lack of a better term, you're out of jail.

Notes on Mark's First Transplant

The improvements in transplant procedures have been so numerous since 2005 that not much of the rest of Mark's experience is relevant to today's transplant candidate. So we will fast-forward.

Mark recovered from the transplant ordeal in two and a half weeks and was released to home recuperation in early July, 2005. In August, he sat Tammy on the back of his Harley and joined his brother, brother-in-law, and their wives on a 4,500 mile-jaunt from Los Angeles to the Annual Sturgis Motorcycle Ralley in Sturgis, South Dakota.

Mark: *The only time I had to push myself was when we went to see the Crazy Horse memorial. My legs were tired. Just one time. Don't know why. We went through temperatures from 114° to 48°. We hit showers coming out of Yellowstone. We were gone for two weeks. I never got sick.*

After we got back, I was ready to go to work but the doctors at UCLA kept me out another six months.

Tammy: *They told us it would take a full year for his immune system to grow back and they didn't want him back in the work routine until he had a working immune system and all his strength.*

The UCLA transplant team released Mark to Dr. Mak in April 2006. Aside from regular check-ups, pieces of normality began falling back into place until February 2008.

Mark: *I had been seeing Dr. Mak every couple of months. He started noticing my hemoglobin count dropping. M-spike going up a bit. I had a series of blood transfusions for anemia.*

February 2008 marked the end of Mark's remission and his return to battle. When remission ends, subtle changes in the disease have taken place. It is henceforth reclassified as *refractory* myeloma and it is treated differently.

The words *remission, relapse,* and *refractory* disease are a few terms used to describe the status of one's disease.

- Remission is used to describe disease that was once present but is no longer detected and an absence of signs and symptoms. It is important to understand that while the signs and symptoms of cancer have disappeared, the cancer may still be in the body—even after treatment. It is not the same as being "cured"; there is no cure for multiple myeloma. During remission, there may be no need for treatment other than supportive care to alleviate any of the ongoing physical effects of the disease or to address any emotional needs. Remission may last a few months or for years. The length of remission depends on the specifics of your individual disease.
- Relapse is used to describe the return of the signs and symptoms of disease following a period of remission or other improvements.
- Refractory disease refers to disease that does not respond to therapy (also called resistant).

It was decided that treatment should aim toward a second transplant, which meant a return to chemotherapy using a particular group of anti-angiogenesis drugs that are most successful in fighting the disease after it has returned: Thalomid, Revlimid, Velcade, Decadron.

Tammy: *Each one worked for a while. Then we'd try something else. Velcade worked particularly well but he got bad neuropathy* (numbness and pain in hands and feet). *We had to go to an acupuncturist for that.*

Mark: *In September 2010, Dr. Vescio told us about Kyprolis* (carfilzomib). *It worked right away. My counts went back to normal. I felt good again.*

Tammy: *It was working so well we stayed on it as a maintenance drug. But our history with other drugs had been that they worked well for a while and then a switch would turn them off. I was afraid it could happen again. I had heard about other patients, including a local doctor, who stayed on maintenance drugs too long. One day—bam!—we would be at a place where [the transplant option would be lost].*

We thought, what the heck, we got two and a half years out of the first transplant. Who knows how much more time we might get out of the next one. We had heard of people getting five, ten years. So we made the decision to go ahead with another transplant. We never considered the possibility of getting no remission at all. Mark: *We harvested stem cells in May 2011. Enough for two transplants. Then we did the transplant in June. New team. New hospital, Cedars-Sinai. New doctor, Dr. Vescio. Nicer patient quarters.*

Today's Transplant Procedure

This begins a general blow-by-blow description of what happens during a transplant. Perhaps it over generalizes. But new patients want candor and simplicity, and we will try to present it.

There were, at the time of this writing, 122 stem cell transplant centers in the United States. Though they are in constant conversation to improve patient care, one cannot presume that because one of them does things one way that any other transplant center does it the exact same way.

Also be reminded that there are two sorts of transplant. The most common is the one in which you have your own stem cells harvested and then returned. There is also the sort in which a donor is found. Both autologous (uses your cells) and allogeneic (donor cells) transplants[16] follow a generally similar path.

---

16 There are also minitransplant procedures. Things happen in the same order for minitransplants but less care is necessary. Precautions to protect from infections are fewer. Sometimes a minitransplant is an outpatient procedure. The patient's body goes through far less stress and discomfort. This is not the preferred treatment strategy for healthy, vigorous patients who can tolerate the full program.

The obvious differences have to do with measures for harvesting your own stem cells for an autologous procedure, versus preparing your body to get somebody else's cells. Your medical team sees great distinctions. So does your insurance company. You will experience about the same number of slings and arrows either way.

The Procedure, Step One—Drugs to Stop Your Myeloma's Aggressive Behavior

You begin by going through a period of chemotherapy that aims to minimize the disease, as Mark Famularo did. (You will recall that these drugs stop the body's blood cell renewal process, which stymies myeloma.) This chemo may reduce your energy and may slightly impact your short-term memory. Early treatments may cause nausea. Later treatments may bring bouts of numbness to hands and feet.

Except for times just after treatments, it may also give you a sense of greater wellness. As Mark concluded during his chemo, *Hey, I can handle this.*

Your anti-angiogenesis chemo will continue until you are ready for step three—mobilization. Meanwhile, step two is added.

Step Two—Tests

Batteries of tests are administered to learn about all your health conditions. The matters of greatest concern are your general ability to deal with physical stress and recover. The good health of your heart, liver, kidneys, and lungs are also measured. These tests predict the success of the transplant. If you don't pass, no transplant. If you do, the transplant is very likely going to be successful. Not a promise, but close.

When the disease minimization process and the test results meet the minimum standards of the transplant team, the procedure date, which had been penciled in, is made firm.

Step Three—Mobilization

This is the autologous (uses your cells) pathway. You skip mobilization if you are prepping for an allogeneic transplant.

Stem cells exist as a percentage of all blood cells. The older you are, the lower the percentage. The strategy during this step is to get your body to produce a maximum amount of myeloma-free blood, thereby maximizing the number of stem cells to be sought and harvested.

If your blood is rich in stem cells, one harvest—called an apheresis, remember?—may be all that's necessary. Those who are more senior can expect to go through more than one of these procedures; you'll find it inconvenient but nothing more than that.

The worst news may be that you are going to lose your hair. Not all mobilization programs make you bald, but many do. Then it grows back. Perhaps thicker than you remember. Perhaps grayer.

The more important matter is that at the start of the mobilization step, your body is still full of malignant myeloma cells. So an atom bomb—Cytoxan or a drug like it—is detonated, destroying your myeloma cells. A lot of healthy white blood cells die in this carnage, too.

Over the next few hours, you will be kept in an antiseptic place while an IV flushes all the dead little critters out of your system. Then you get a blood transfusion and go home, where you will rest and do your best to stay clean and sterile.[17]

Back in the hospital a few days later, Neupogen, a *growth factor* also known as G-CSF, is injected. This accelerates the production of fresh, myeloma-free bone marrow.

In as short a time as a day, your body will produce a decent supply of blood from which stem cells for your transplant can be harvested. You'll need a few million. One little bag full.

---

17 See Health Tips, p.136

If practical, enough for two or more transplants will be harvested. Several rounds of the drugs-then-apheresis cycle may be necessary.

Be patient with this process. During his second time through this, Mark Famularo went through seven daily Neupogen injections, followed by five harvest days. Out of that, he got enough cells for his transplant, plus—very fortunately—one extra dose to bank.

And then he rested at home, and so will you.

Step Four—Conditioning

On June 1, 2011, Mark Famularo checked into Cedars Sinai's transplant unit. They took some blood for lab tests. Checked his vitals. Installed an IV and with one *push* of melphalan from a syringe into his saline drip solution, began the process of killing the cancer. He rested until the next morning and then received the second half of his melphalan.

Tammy: *They gave him a mouth full of ice chips before the melphalan, and that kept it from getting to the nerve endings in his throat and mouth, causing boils ... I don't think he had any sores that time ... it was (generally) much easier on him physically.*

Melphalan makes the patient nauseated and weak. Pain in bones and joints is common. Several days of feeling lousy follow while the melphalan hunts down and eradicates myeloma cells. The patient has no appetite; will need help and encouragement to get out of bed; will be dull and listless; and will need pain meds.

Tammy: *You have to be there for your patient. You have to be the advocate and helper as much as you can. He was so weak and sick there was no way he could get everything he needed. The nurses were great but they had other patients ... they're all overworked.*

Truthfully, I can't imagine having to go through this without a caregiver. But I know that people do. And, [as a caregiver,] I feel good that by my being there, the nurses could spend more time with those patients.

Step Five—Transplant

Two days after conditioning, the melphalan has done its job. New, healthy stem cells are given by IV. Often with some ceremony.

Shortly, perhaps within a day, you notice feeling better. Your blood counts, which were at ridiculously low levels after the melphalan, begin to improve. These are signals that the little colony of healthy bone marrow has dug in and is growing. By your new birthday plus 10 to 20 days, your platelet count should be high enough to keep you from bouts of spontaneous bleeding. Your red cells, though still showing that you are anemic, increase daily. Your growing white cell counts show that your immune system is functioning and growing stronger.

You go home. You observe sanitary and dietary rules and you get better. Aside from post-transplant check-ups and perhaps blood transfusions, and a maintenance drug or two, you get your life back.

Plan B

Step five was how it is supposed to happen; how it happens nine times out of 10. In Mark Famularo's case, the blood counts came back, but so did the myeloma.

Mark: *We knew within two months that the second transplant didn't take.*

Tammy: *Your blood counts have to be at a certain level before you achieve remission. We got close but never there. So Doc Vescio said, what do you want to do? And we decided on a carfilzomib (Kyprolis) clinical trial.*

Mark: *(Five months later) ... around December 2011, I started developing a tumor on my forehead. About May 2012, they decided to stop the carfilzomib because of the tumor. Later they did a PET scan and discovered there were several of them.*

Tammy: *Sometimes you have to game the system in a clinical trial. In this case, the tumor was disturbing but we thought the carfilzomib was doing its job as a maintenance drug. We all knew that if we reported the tumor, they'd take the carfilzomib away. So we tried things to treat the tumor and sort of ignored it officially. You do things like that to keep as much of the system working for you as possible.*

For the next three months Mark went on Treanda (bendamustine). [18]

Mark: *Right now Treanda seems to be working very well ... We have decisions to make. It may be that it will work for a long time but that is not our experience with new drugs.*

Tammy: *When it was clear that the last transplant was not going to work, Dr. Vescio suggested we move toward a tandem transplant; one transplant using Mark's stem cells, followed by a second transplant with donor cells.*

You have to begin with chemo, and it has to work for three months. Bendamustine is working for Mark, so that fits the plan. Then they put him in the hospital for an autologous transplant using the cells we already have banked. Two months later we do a donor transplant.

The Chapter Closes

It is time for you to take the lessons of Mark and Tammy's experiences and to apply those that relate to the road before you. As you go, know that they

---

18 This is the lead drug in a treatment protocol. Decadron is also part of this treatment.

gave of themselves in this chapter as their gift to you.

Tips for the Transplant Patient

Mark: *Think about yourself. You may be a parent or the breadwinner and used to putting everybody else first. This is a time when that focus should change. Stay within yourself. Focus on your illness. If I don't feel like doing something I just don't do it.*

Start a blog or appoint someone to be your spokesman to tell those who need to know how you're doing.

Chew ice chips during the melphalan. Cram your mouth full.

During the conditioning step, the smell of food is nauseating.

I also had pain in my bones: arms, legs, back, joints. Cushions helped me.

I got cold. Had shakes. Get blankets from the nurses.

Force yourself up. Walk the halls. You'll get home sooner.

Take a minimum amount of medicine for discomfort. Strong pain medicine causes severe constipation and other complications. The medical staff will tend to be too generous with pain meds.

You won't have much energy for computers and that sort of thing. After the melphalan you're not good for much more than TV. You want to be left alone to vegetate. I took a two-DVD set that I wanted to watch. ESPN has this program they call "30 for 30." Thirty shows. One hour each. I watched three of them.

Look forward to things that will make you feel better. For me it was going home. Familiar surroundings. And I wanted a mustard hot dog. When I got home and Tam fixed me that hot dog, it tasted sooo good.

Know your limits. Tammy made me two of them. I could only eat one.

Once you are home, set small goals. One of mine was to walk up the stairs.

You need someone special to be with you. I don't know how I would have gotten through this without Tammy. (She's always had my back.) ... [W]hen we're at the doctor's, she'll think of things to ask about that I don't.

These drugs can depress you. Without her, I don't know how I would have gone on.

I have programmed myself to get by things in steps. Right now I want to get past the recovery from the last (second) transplant attempt. Then the next transplants. Then I want to get back to normal. Get back to work. Restart my career.

Tammy: *Encourage people who want to see you to wait until you get home after the transplant. People would drive a long way. Pay to park. And Mark would feel obligated to visit with them. Lots of times, he just wasn't ready for that. He was so tired.*

(Look past the long treatment road ahead.) *Set goals. Our daughter wants us to go to Italy ... She and her husband want to go and I would like us to go with them. But mainly I want Mark to recover so he's around when our daughter starts having kids.*

Tips for the Transplant Patient's Caregiver

Tammy: *The Caring Bridge* (caringbridge.org) *has been a godsend for me. It was organized so I could use it immediately. Photos. Message center—people go in there and send us messages.Reports on how Mark is doing. There's a guest book and his story; how he was diagnosed and all that. Anybody who cares about us can go there any time.*

The nurse's station stocks a lot of things your patient needs for comfort—lotion, booties, ChapStick, other things. Go ask for what you need.

He'd get crabby. I learned to not let him get away with it.

One thing I would tell a new caregiver watching someone go through this—if you get depressed, go see someone about it.

The other thing is to take care of yourself. Stay healthy. You can't be a cheerleader if you aren't up to it.

You've got to keep living with it but you can't let this disease run your life ... or you don't have a life.

The Day After Tomorrow

If "Bones" McCoy, chief medical officer, Starship Enterprise, is right, these treatments for myeloma will be thought of as barbaric, sometime in the future. The defenders of the United Federation of Planets in the year 2373 will have left all treatment discomfort and uncertainty behind.

But that is Hollywood wishful thinking and this is how it is.

Valley of the Shadow

Part of you belongs to me now,

A gift, freely given

But still not easy

Not for you, the donor, nor for me, the recipient

My own bone marrow beaten into submission

First by disease and then by treatment
So your gift could bring me new life
Spirit and soul have been repaired
Now I have hope,
A new person,
But not just inside my bones
My transplant from you carries also
A bit of your soul,
So we are now brothers
We've journeyed together
Through the valley of the shadow
Neither will ever be the same
Both of us given a gift
—Malin Dollinger, MD

16

Thoughts on the Human Condition: Sometimes Things Go Wrong

Jim Tamkin, MD

We strive for perfection knowing that our best is not always good enough.

Despite everyone's best intentions, things can go wrong. This is not a prediction that anything *will* go wrong. But I think it is in every myeloma patient's best interest to be prepared. Pay attention and learn as much as possible about what your medical teams are up to, and why. Think about common sense contributions you can make to avoid complications.

An Illustration

Just a week before beginning work on this chapter, my kidneys were acting up and I was hospitalized. Kidney failure begets dialysis. So there I was, in nothing but a thin patient gown, in a room with the thermostat set at 66 degrees. My teeth began to chatter, to which the attending technician commented,

"Being cold is pretty common in here." My caregiver, and wife these past 46 years, asked him to get me a blanket. Ten or 15 minutes later word came back that there were no blankets. I am now shaking violently and reasonably certain of pneumonia.

My wife takes charge. Ignoring the stares of the staff, she locates the supply closet and searches it. When no blanket is found, she goes down the hall, comes back with two blankets and a glare that spoke volumes. This is a hospital. You don't run out of blankets. Elapsed time: Maybe two minutes.

"Do you know why they keep that room at 66 degrees?" she asked me later.

I presumed it was to keep the equipment at optimum operating temperature. "Oh no!" she tells me. "It's for the comfort of the staff. They wear hospital uniforms over their street clothes, which makes them warm. So they crank up the A/C."

This is a true story. But it is not a condemnation. The supply closet in the dialysis room is normally well stocked and the people who work the room are usually more considerate. The point is that my caregiver used her head when others in the room forgot to use theirs and the patient benefited. You may need to do likewise.

Mistakes and Omissions

Med school, like all boot camps, intends to beat the recruits into a mindset that does not tolerate sloth or mistake. Regardless of the circumstances, the problem-solving process continues in a focused and dedicated manner until the patient's needs have been met.

Other members of medical teams, nurses in particular, learn this mindset equally well.

Mistakes, omissions, poor choices, miscommunications, and ignorance never stop trying to confound treatment. We know that they are in the room when our patients are before us. We go to extraordinary measures to remove them from the equation so that they don't compromise our best efforts.

But they are always, always there.

You will encounter these foibles. You will want to blame someone, which may be appropriate. But understand that this is, at root, our human condition seeping out, exacerbated by our very complicated and very serious disease.

On the positive side, your act of realizing that a mistake has been made is personally valuable. It permits growth, improving your effectiveness as a proactive patient or caregiver.

Keep Your Cool

Medicine, when taught in the classroom, or when practiced anywhere that understanding and optimism prevail, should have a very good result. Fortunately, that is most of the time.

But the reason you are reading these words has to do with an impatient, uncomfortable, remorseless cancer that we don't know enough about yet. It is complicated. The treatments for it can have toxic side effects. Emergency treatment conditions result.

When there's no time for calm consideration, everybody tends to go into crisis mode—the docs, the nurses, the techs, the receptionist, and the security guard—and you. Know it now and it will help when you find yourself in a treatment situation that demands a cool head and creativity.

Keep Your Eye on the Ball

Sometime before kindergarten, we get introduced to the game of catch. Mom or dad shows you the ball and then gently lofts it toward your outstretched hands. After a few tries, you catch it. The basic lesson—keep your eye on the ball—is taught in every culture I know of, and I've seen more of the world than most.

Like other symptoms of the human condition, we sometimes forget to keep our eye on the ball when it really matters. Take, as a pointed example, another recent hospital stay of mine. My story begins at 3a.m.

A nurse woke me. "Time for your medication."

Me: "Uhhh ... Oh, hi. What medicine is that?"

Nurse: "It's for your high blood pressure."

Me: "But I have normal blood pressure."

Nurse: "This is on your chart. Doctor's orders."

Me: "Why should I take medicine to reduce my normal blood pressure?"

Nurse, nearing the end of a long shift and somewhat exasperated: "Are you refusing to take your medicine?"

I knew that if I took that pill, I might end up in intensive care, instead of being discharged a few hours later. Worst case, I could become 1 of the 195,000 American hospital patients who die each year due to hospital error.[19] I also knew that my nurse was not in his best professional frame of mind. He was going about his duties without thinking; his eye was not on the ball.

---

19 A n average of 195,000 Americans died annually in 2000, 2001, and 2002 because of potentially preventable, in-hospital medical errors, according to a study of 37 million patient records by HealthGrades, a health care quality company.

So what happens when you, neither a physician nor conversant with the potential effects of the wrong medicine, are confronted by a nurse in the middle of the night?

To begin with, you'd better know enough about your status to participate in the discussion. It is standard hospital practice for patients to be carefully briefed on their condition, its treatments, and schedules at a time when everyone is fully alert. All patients and caregivers need do is pay attention.

"That happened to me," Pat Killingsworth told his Stillwater, Minnesota, myeloma support group. Pat, a myeloma patient who had just celebrated 44 months of high-quality survival after diagnosis, was in a clinic. The staff wanted to give him a shot to *boost* the count of a blood element that was *not low.*

"I don't think I need that," he said.

The nurse gave one of those impatient looks we've all seen, a heightened eyebrow and that set jaw that says your condition needs this needle full of stuff, so cut the palaver and roll up that sleeve.

"I caved," Killingsworth said. "I took the shot. Then didn't feel my best for the next couple of days ... It's tough. Looking back on it, I knew the shot was probably not right for me. I should have asked for verification from my doc."

It's really easy for Monday morning quarterbacks to say *Yeah, Pat, you should have.* Our affliction is poorly understood and deadly serious. And I have to say that, of all the things we should do with unerring accuracy, one of the toughest is to stop busy professionals when things don't ring true, to ask what may well be a stupid question, and not to care if it is.

Returning to my 3a.m. encounter with the wrong pill, I asked my nurse to summon his shift supervisor. The three of us examined my chart and reasoned together. The happy consensus was that I should not take the pill.

Keep Clean

Myeloma and its treatments have compromised our immune systems. It is easier for us to pick up new illnesses and infections.

- Wash your hands frequently. Insist that those who visit you—and hospital staff—do the same. Don't allow any opportunity for contagion to spread.
- When you are hospitalized, you are in a very vulnerable place. There are lots of ways your condition can be complicated by the illnesses of other patients and the microbes naturally resident there.

    * If blood is drawn, be certain that any spill is immediately cleaned up. Blood out of the body encourages all manner of infection.

* The same is obviously true of other bodily fluids, notably urine and feces.

* Spilled IV fluids must also be thoroughly scrubbed up.

* General room cleanliness is essential. Remains of meals must go. Cut flowers, now wilted, may be dangerous. Drinks, candy wrappers, newspapers, and other things that visitors leave in the room must be disposed of.

* When food servers bring meals to you, expect that they will be practicing sterile procedures. If they do not, don't touch the food.

- Remind visitors to keep their contagious diseases, even colds, to themselves. Youthful visitors are embodiments of Typhoid Mary, with playground and classroom viruses by the bushel. Love them from a distance.

"My husband, Gary, needed a catheter implanted near his spine to transport a tumor shrinking treatment. His physician rushed in to perform a procedure that he obviously felt pressured by time to complete quickly.

In his haste, he didn't don surgical gloves, which surprised me. I should have said something. But the hurry-hurry-hurry mood in the room, his exalted hospital rank and intimidating demeanor froze me.

In minutes the catheter was implanted and he was gone. The result was that Gary's incision became infected. I spent the last year of Gary's life treating a weeping wound that wouldn't heal."

—Anita Chambers

Ask Around Until You're Sure

You may have never met an oncologist, and that may be fine. But the medical community in general expects physicians in other specialties to refer myeloma patients—not just to oncologists, cancer doctors, but to specialists within oncology. If that has not been your experience, please learn the reason from your physician.

It is very common for myeloma diagnosis to be carried even further. In my case, five physicians I knew by reputation each gave me an independent evaluation. It may also interest you to know that they disagreed as to what I should do. Though either of the paths that these experts recommended may have been good, I had to listen, learn, decide, and take responsibility for the outcome.

Those who were diagnosed some time ago and are now in established treatment protocols may be past the time when supporting examinations and testing have value. Options have come and gone, and a path is set. But recently diagnosed patients who have not obtained second opinions and perhaps don't know their options have some work to do. After 10-plus years since my initial tests and recommendations, I am living proof that multiple evaluations and informed planning would be a good idea for you.

Possible Impediments to Best Care

I believe that everyone has a right to the best health care possible. Period. No exceptions. There are other points of view.

- A growing number argue that limitations ought to be imposed. The planet is overcrowded. A person who has lived to age 65 or maybe 75 has lived a good long time. Perhaps we should not make quite as many heroic efforts to preserve such a life as we might if the person were 25.
- I have colleagues who would accept a spending limit of $100,000 per year on the health of a person. A myeloma patient receiving a stem cell transplant can romp through a number that low in a month. On an annual basis, myeloma may be the most costly form of cancer to treat; most costly when all the procedures and drugs are totaled; most costly to the patient, even after all the health insurance and discounts have been applied.

- There are those, too, who look at the cost of our medical care and see a greater global need. The money spent on a stem cell transplant might buy enough vaccine to inoculate an entire region, saving hundreds or even thousands of lives.
- There are also physicians, and others in the healing arts, who may not give a 100% effort to the health needs of the incurably ill. Not many. But a few. In most cases, these are people who have yet to face a stricken mother, father, wife, husband, son, or daughter.
- Certainly, *death panel* is too harsh, but there are committees in both health care agencies and insurance companies that decide who gets care now and who must wait, or jump through extra administrative and economic hoops. They've established requirements that have nothing to do with doctors caring for patients. Similar thinking has already traumatized health care in big parts of Europe.

Of all the human conditions, the urge to over legislate the ways we save the lives of very sick people is one of the easiest to understand—and one of the most pernicious. Myeloma patients—who are often senior citizens, and who fight an implacable foe—are likely to face a serious questioner of one of these sorts. It is important to be thoughtful in reply to their concerns.

My ethical standard urges me to do the very best I can to preserve my health and to prolong my life. My ethical standard urges me to urge you to do likewise. Those who tell us that we are too old, or too sick, or less worthy than some others to receive the very best that the healing arts have to offer are wrong.

Ignorance

Speaking of human conditions, one cannot hang around oncology long without encountering patients and caregivers who do not know the type of cancer they face, cannot say what medicine they are taking, and profess similar ignorance on other core issues. Such people are wire-walking without a net.

Our nation's hospitals spend extraordinary sums of money to have qualified translators on hand for those who struggle with English. We have counselors representing every faith. A new patient with linguistic or ethical issues can be helped.

We also encounter those who have not exercised their intellectual skills in some time and others with various mind sets that make an understanding of our disease and its treatments difficult. You are not among them. You would not be reading this if you were.

Where you see ignorance, lovingly but urgently encourage understanding.

The Bureaucracy

> *This battleship has gone through wars ... but never through the bureaucracy.*
>
> *—Los Angeles City Councilwoman Janice Hahn, on the frustrations associated with getting the Navy to park the mothballed battleship USS Iowa in the LA Harbor as a museum*

There are numerous jibes at our bureaucratic institutions. My favorite: You were not among those authorized to initial this memo. Please erase your initials and initial the erasure.

American bureaucrats are rated tops of all the organizational men and women in the world. Even so, when given health care to manage, they give us more to fear than fear itself. This is not a political statement. It is the cry of a guy whose affairs have been haunted by the best intentions of massive organizations since my days as a Navy public health services doctor, trying to protect the well-being of Arizona's Cocopah and Quechan Indians, 40 years ago, at the Ft. Yuma Hospital.

I urge you to maintain a respectful concern for the ways that our insurance companies, our hospitals, HMOs, welfare agencies, nonprofits, and other large institutions plan to deal with us. Things never go exactly right. We can also hope that things never go exactly wrong.

Some of these recommendations have been mentioned earlier, but they are so important I cannot emphasize them enough:

- Keep a chronological record in a notebook. Record the names, titles, responsibilities, address, and phone numbers of those who serve you. Write down the gist of every key fact you are told, and by whom. Note dates that prescriptions are filled and by which pharmacy.
- Keep a calendar for upcoming events. It may be helpful to include medications you take and to check off daily doses as you take them.
- Demand a copy of every piece of paper generated by your health team and all those third parties in the bureaucracy: Every test, prescription, admission, discharge, diagnosis, authorization, notification. Ask for film, CDs, and DVDs after imaging, surgical procedures, and at any other time digital recordkeeping is evident.

There are administrators and nurses who will suggest that some of these records are *confidential,* or for some other reason may not be given to you. They are incorrect. You owned that information the moment someone put your name on it. Demand them. A small copying fee is sometimes charged.

- If you don't know why some form is given to you to complete, ask.
- Carefully consider the consequences before granting bureaucrats permission to share your records with third parties. Ask for a good reason to say yes. There are often good reasons to say no.
- When those serving you ask for permission to discard some of your records, say no. You, a medical specialist you haven't met yet, your attorney, or your estate, may need something later.

17

Is It Too Late for Broccoli? The Role of Diet and Herbs

> *Let food be your medicine and medicine be your food.*
>
> —*Hippocrates, 460–370BC*

Take an integrative approach to fighting myeloma.

> *I totally believe in a team-based approach. If the patient doesn't have good support in all areas of health management, he can't benefit fully from conventional treatment. We have to move integrated medicine from second place to first place for myeloma patients.*
>
> —*Mary L. Hardy, MD*
> *Medical Director*
> *Simms/Mann – UCLA Center for Integrative Oncology*
> *July 23, 2009*

There is a direct line of descent from Hippocrates' thinking to Dr. Hardy's. Everything in life should be integrated into the healing process. Why else, when none of it is covered by insurance, would cancer patients lay out an estimated $28 billion a year for "holistic spiritual practice and physical exercise, as well as vitamin and herbal medicines for enhanced tumoricidal (sic) activity or reduction in treatment-related adverse events?" We have to combine the best practices of conventional and complementary medicine.

The approach has some impressive advocates. The Block Center for Integrative Cancer Treatment, Evanston, Illinois, claims a very high treatment success rate for cancer patients.

> *If only cancer were easily cured with a single therapy. But the magic bullet approach to treating disease is generally more myth than fact. Truly effective treatment requires innovative thinking and a multi-faceted approach.*
>
> *In the case of cancer, the tumor itself is only part of the problem. Conditions surrounding the tumor and its environment must be changed.... For this reason we modify what we refer to as the "biochemical terrain" while focusing on the whole person, not simply the disease.*
>
> *Keith I. Block, MD*
> *Medical-Scientific Director*
>
> *Penny B. Block, PhD*
> *Executive Director*

Botanical Medicine

Dr. Hardy's special interest is in botanical medicine, having trained with scientists and herbalists from China, Peru, the Amazon, Kenya, and South Africa.

Conventional treatment wisdom, she says, generally recommends complete avoidance of all dietary supplements, especially during chemotherapy and radiation. This doctor-directed interdiction is often ignored by patients, who continue to take vitamins and eat foods they find most satisfying on the sly.

Sometimes patients harm themselves through this self-medication, but more often the food supplements help, Dr. Hardy believes. Physicians running conventional treatment programs notice these unexplained good results and can't account for them. It would be so much better for patient and physician if an integrated approach to treatment were open on the table.

Dr. Hardy begins her first interview with a new patient by explaining the process she uses for healing. It is a team approach in which she brings in experts in both conventional and alternative medicine to use as she and the patient feel is necessary.

Common sense is your friend, she tells them. Sometimes half the medicines the patient was taking before coming to Dr. Hardy immediately go in the trash.

Based on individual diagnostics, Dr. Hardy creates a plan tailored specifically to the patient. The following is for illustrative purposes only, but describes the type of regimen most of her patients begin, including:

- Four or five small meals a day
- Lots of cabbage and mustard greens
- Protein with every meal: Beans, tofu, whey products, fish, chicken, eggs
- Monounsaturated fats, including olive oil and fish oils
- Limited dairy and meat (but not eliminated)
- Vitamins C[20] and D

For specifics and menus, Dr. Hardy suggests consulting with a nutritionist specializing in help for cancer patients who are in treatment.

What You Need to Know About the FDA and Regulation

Ancient civilizations relied on medical observation to identify herbs, drugs, and therapies that worked, and those that did not. Beginning in the early 20th century, physicians and pharmacists began to develop

---

20 If you are in active chemotherapy, high-dose vitamin C is incompatible with Velcade (bortezomib).

the concept of the *well-controlled* therapeutic drug trial. A worldwide drug disaster in 1961[21] resulted in the enactment of the 1962 Drug Amendments, which explicitly stated that the Food and Drug Administration (FDA) would rely on scientific testing and that new drug approvals would be based not only upon proof of safety, but also on *substantial evidence* that the drug worked.

This vastly increased bureaucratic manpower and quickly led to a confrontation between federal government scientists and the naturopathic industry selling traditional herbs and teas. The feds wanted every twig and seed put through the same rigorous lab work and clinical trial processes that the pharmaceutical industry's products faced.

Millions of Americans with cultural ties to traditional healing products objected. They knew that products they relied on would instantly vanish from store shelves. Grandma's cellar stash would make her a criminal. Then, when the stuff had jumped through all the government hoops, it was certain to come back on the market at 10 times higher price.

The world's herbal medicinal industry was also horrified. It had been selling products whose only guarantees—if any—had to do with where the product had been dug up or picked, and any measures taken

---

21 Thalidomide was found to have caused several tens of thousands of birth defects.

to ensure purity. Patient safety was generally thought of as the responsibility of the person administering the item, and—truth be told—it really wasn't a concern. China alone had more than 16,000 herbal products in therapeutic use. Applying FDA standards to each of them would require hundreds of years and bankrupt the world.

A compromise was struck. Any *natural* product on the market before 1964 could continue to be sold—so long as it remained in the same form. Moreover, it could not be found to be harmful to health or to be intoxicating. This judgment was and is a lawyer's delight. As an example, if one takes oolong tea, a pre-1964 product, and blends it with orange pekoe tea, another pre-1964 product, must the FDA pass judgment?

We face a real quandary, with neither the boys in the lab coats nor the witch doctors they warn us about looking wholly ethical and impartial.

On the one hand:

Since the 1994 passage of the Dietary Supplement Health and Education Act, which created today's regulatory framework, the number of natural compounds on the market has shot from 4,000 to 55,000. Meanwhile the FDA has received what it terms *adequate notification* for 170 of them.

On the other hand:

A 2010 study sponsored by the National Cancer Institute of the National Institutes of Health discovered that mice with colon cancer, who had become nauseated after chemotherapy, were relieved by PHY906, a compound that the FDA considers experimental.

PHY906, also known as Huang Qin Tang, is a formulation of licorice, peony blossom, skullcap, and jujube that physicians in Asia have been using to treat nausea, vomiting, cramping, and diarrhea for 1,800 years.

FDA approval of PHY960 is still pending, but researchers such as Cathy Eng, the Department of Gastrointestinal Medical Oncology, M.D. Anderson Cancer Center in Houston, encourage the FDA to finish its examination so that 21st-century America can, in the opinion of naturopathic medicine, catch up.

The National Center for Complementary and Alternative Medicine

The federal government's National Institutes of Health (NIH) has 27 arms. One of them is the National Cancer Institute. Another is the National Center for Complementary and Alternative Medicine. They are co-equal on the NIH organizational chart—meaning that the two pursuits of medicine are peers—even though the cancer institute is many times the size of the complementary and alternative treatments group.

Perhaps this means that science fully respects the smaller endeavor but has not yet seen all the ways it will one day contribute to our welfare and happiness.

The Consensus

Complementary and alternative medicines are real and potent. They are also often misused and abused. Mainstream medicine has the same issues. Of the several dozen authoritative voices who have contributed to this discussion, the consensus is that:

- A thoughtful blend of styles and healing tools is the most comfortable palette for most myeloma treatment teams.
- It is at least dangerous and most likely tragic to use alternative medications and techniques *in place of* conventional medicine.
- There is a whole lot going on here that nobody understands.

18

Pain Management Coping Tools

Pain management is an essential skill.

As a myeloma patient, you can experience various sorts of discomfort without warning—feelings ranging from numbness to achiness to sharp, throbbing pain. Successful pain management, the process by which you overcome these feelings, is essential.

You have choices as to how you go about this, and who you go to for help.

The Complexity of Discomfort

Pain and numbness have multiple causes. As pain manager, you need to have a good idea of where the sensation is coming from and what caused it. You should also have some idea of how tough your adversary is going to be. Some pains can be relieved with aspirin or Tylenol. Some can't. Some numbness responds to medication. Some may require radiation or surgery. Sometimes an acupuncturist or other specialized health practitioner may be most effective.

None of this is simple. You must evaluate your discomforts in a precise, orderly way. You are building an arsenal of weapons to counter an array of attackers. It will probably seem overwhelming at first. That will pass. But you're never going to bat 1,000. Sensations will come out of nowhere to bedevil and irritate both you and your medical team. Sometimes solutions you once relied on will stop working or begin producing an unwanted side effect, like an allergic rash or a gastrointestinal problem.

In the Beginning

The sorts of pains and their location are largely dependent on your form of myeloma and on its stage or status. Other pains come from secondary sources. You broke a bone. A tooth needs filling. Another, unrelated physical condition like diabetes or inflammatory bowel disease is demanding your attention. Pain management has to be something that you and your doctor—or the specialist brought in to consult on this matter—specifically designs for you with all the contingencies considered. So listen closely to your *painmeister* and when you are at home, carefully treat your pain within the boundaries that your med team has set for you.

Pills and Shots

When you think of pain management, you probably think of pills, possibly augmented by shots. This is a generally accurate picture for many people, though sometimes complicated when other pills and shots are needed to counter the adverse side effects of the first bunch.

Radiation as Pain Killer

A pocket of myeloma may form somewhere without you or the doc realizing. It becomes painful. Your team uses measures that worked in the past and wonder why the pain's still there. Then imaging reveals the tumor. Mystery solved. Your radiation oncologist zaps it. Immediate relief.

Surgery as Pain Killer

Tumors on or inside bones are sometimes best removed by surgery.

Loss of bone mass, because of myeloma or a drug side effect, can be fixed by reinforcement.

If you ever need an incentive to be super diligent in your treatment regimen, these reinforcing surgeries, notably vertebroplasty or kyphoplasty[22]—required after myeloma has destroyed backbone integrity—provide it. You do not want to let your disease present you with problems of this sort.

---

22 These procedures use cement to mend structural loss of the spine.

Complementary Therapies

If your cultural heritage is Asian or East Asian, or Native American, you may view Western medicine with some caution. The simplistic way that this chapter's opening sections leapt to management through pills, radiation, and surgery may have struck you as less likely the path to wellness than the diagnosis and treatment customs of your forbearers.

More and more oncology treatment teams, though still Western in basic mind set, are looking East. Gary Deng, MD, PhD, is a physician–scientist on the Integrative Medicine Service at Memorial Sloan-Kettering Cancer Center. He is a board-certified internist and acupuncturist with clinical interests in symptom control, supportive care, and health maintenance in cancer patients and cancer survivors. Dr. Deng received his medical degree from Beijing Medical University, in China, and his PhD in microbiology and immunology from the University of Miami, in Florida. He is the principal investigator or co-principal investigator of several symptom control and botanical research projects. He has authored review articles on integrative medicine and textbook chapters in *Cancer Medicine, Internal Medicine Care of Cancer Patients, Principle and Practice of Palliative and Supportive Oncology,* and *PDQ Integrative Oncology.*

Dr. Deng advises us that a diverse group of treatment therapies may offer greater pain management effectiveness.

Dietary Supplements and Herbs

Some natural herbs, vitamins, minerals, and plants are effective pain, stress, and nausea fighters. Memorial Sloan-Kettering created databases and commentary on its website at www.mskcc.org for review of this area of Asian experience, some of which goes back two or three thousand years. These medicines can bebiologically active, having both effects and side effects.

Mind–Body Medicines

Reiki therapy from Japan, aroma therapies from India, and Western music therapy are notable methods of harnessing the power of links between mind and body to promote pain control and healing.

According to Deng, music therapy is being used a lot in palliative care, as "music touches a deep part of our soul." In his experience, it reduces suffering in patients with very advanced disease.

Body-Based Practices

Touch therapy is a major part of what Deng offers to patients with aches and pains and tension. He explains that touch therapy tends to reduce chronic wear and tear or muscle strains and reduces anxiety. He uses several different techniques such as Swedish massage, reflexology focused on the feet, and Shiatsu (massage) from Japan.

Acupuncture

Deng acknowledges that there is good evidence supporting acupuncture in controlling chronic pain, but the success of acupuncture is highly dependent on the skill of the healer. In some patients, if the practitioners are not well-trained, there could be harm. According to Deng, in rare instances patients with immune suppression or bleeding tendencies are harmed by acupuncture. So the choice of a good acupuncturist is very important.

Focused Attention Meditation

One of the oldest, and many believe most effective, ways to control pain is known as focused attention meditation. According to a 2011 study published in *The Journal of Neuroscience,* redirecting pain sensations using focused breathing may reduce pain intensity by half and pain unpleasantness by two-thirds.[23] Although this method requires time to train the brain, it is often mastered without the

23 Famously successful pain control technique women use during childbirth: Breathe! Breathe!

coaching of a professional ... though if you need help, your medical team knows where to direct you.

It's good mental exercise, healthy, drug-free, no side effects, available whenever and wherever needed. And there's no co-pay.

Drug Addiction

Most needy patients apparently benefit from highly addictive drugs such as morphine and hydrocodone without becoming junkies. The relief they feel comes without physical dependency. As the medical team's success reduces the pain, the patient's dose of pain medicine is reduced. The body does not overly enjoy the drug's inebriating effect or crave more.

That's the official line, anyway. It does not take related matters into consideration, such as drug experimentation by other members of the family and the mistake recovered patients make by saving an unused portion that is abused later. There are those, too, who consciously or subconsciously welcome inebriation. Medicine's best intentions will have difficulty keeping them sober.

Bottom line: Take the drugs. You've got an illness that is trying to kill you. Worry tomorrow—after pain management has helped your treatment program bring you that glorious dawn.

Pain Med Terms

When your doctor says to you that, *"Any 'n-sayd' is fine"* or *"You won't need an adjuvant with your Vicodin,"* it may help to take a peek at this short list of definitions.

Adjuvant	It's anything they give you that encourages the primary thing you're getting to be effective:
	This kid is running with the football.
	A guy in the stands is beating on the woman in front of him, screaming, Go! Go!
	Hey, that's my wife, growls the man beside her.
	That's my son with the ball! screams the beater.
	Hit her again! shouts the husband.
	Adjuvant football.
Analgesic	Pain reducing
Antipyretic	Fever reducing
Hyperalgesia	An increased sensitivity to pain. Sometimes a powerful pain killer reverses action and heightens the discomfort.
Immune system	Several interacting, highly complex systems within the body that protect against viruses and other invaders.

Metabolism	The breaking down of carbohydrates, proteins, and fats into smaller units; reorganizing those units as tissue building blocks or as energy sources; and eliminating waste products of the processes.
NSAID Pronounced "n-sayd"	All scientific endeavors must have acronyms and this one is a beauty: Nonsteroidal anti-inflammatory drug. It refers to our most common pain killers, such as aspirin, ibuprofen, and naproxen.
Opioid	The first opioid came from the opium poppy. Technically, opioids work by decreasing the perception of pain. Side effects include sedation, respiratory depression, constipation, and a strong sense of euphoria.
	There are natural, synthetic, and semisynthetic opioids.
Palliative	Meant to reduce the suffering of patients. Has no direct role in healing.
Tricyclic antidepressants	Tricyclic and tetracyclic antidepressants affect brain chemicals to ease depression symptoms. These are tools of the psychiatric trade.

World Health Organization Guidelines

You may have wondered who came up with the idea of the 10 faces on the wall of your oncologist's examination room with expression graduating from vapid to wretched.

Nurse: "And how are you feeling today?"

You: "Ehhh, not so great."

Nurse: "So tell me, which of the faces on the chart is most like the way you feel right now?"

You (thinking): "Gosh, there's got to be a more precise way to measure how I feel. They've got super sophisticated tools for everything else..."

It turns out that Los Angeles and Timbuktu have the pain cartoon diagnosing system in common, promulgated by the World Health Organization.

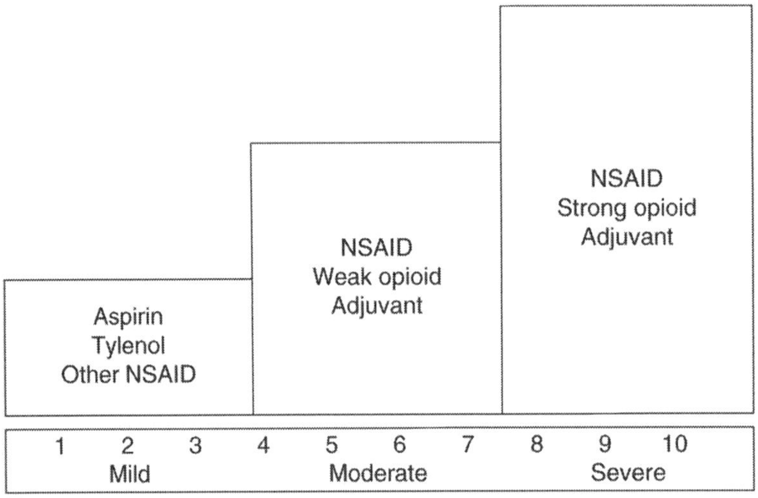

The goal of pain relief is to keep the patient's discomfort down to level 4 or lower, while controlling production of toxic side effects such as delirium, confusion, constipation, nausea, allergies, and rashes.

So, pick the level of your pain from the row of cartoon faces and the chart tells what to do about it.

Mild Pain

Take an aspirin or a Tylenol. Celebrex is also good.

Moderate Pain

NSAID plus a weak narcotic—Vicodin, Lortab, Percocet, Percodan, or OxyContin.

Severe Pain

NSAID plus morphine, Demerol, Dilaudid, fentanyl, or methadone.

Adjuvants

Medications for moderate to severe pain often work more effectively when accompanied by steroids, antidepressants, antihistamines, and sedatives.

Your Pain Control

The WHO guidelines only apply to you in the broadest, most general of senses. Your cancer makes you a much more complicated case than most, and the situation is made even more challenging by your chemo and other drug interactions, co-morbidities (see Chapter 20), and the aging process.

19

Home Care: You'll Visit Hospitals but You'll Live at Home

Home is where the health is.

Consider the Possibilities

If you are a newly diagnosed myeloma patient, there is a good possibility that it will be years—if ever—before your cancer forces you to think about a drastic alteration to your lifestyle. That said, this is the very best time to look at the alternatives and to make plans.

Where Does a Person Go to Be Sick?

The tradition in most cultures is that families take care of their own. Adult children or other relatives open their homes to loved ones needing assistance. This is almost never a seamless, friction-free solution. The chance that it will remain completely harmonious vanishes the day the sick person moves in. Unintended economics and time demands also burden these arrangements. It is still an excellent solution and one with many rewards to the family that makes it work.

There are several sorts of commercial enterprises that offer facilities and staff for those who need long-term care. Some churches and community nonprofits have places; usually for those who are indigent, and often with a time limit.

Major Factors

Support Equipment

A remarkable pile of stuff—from hospital bed, through wheelchair, bedpan to nursing supplies, pill bottles, and orthopedics of one sort or another—accumulates wherever sick people are. The tab to buy or rent it all would knock your hat off if health insurance, nonprofits, and government programs didn't pay for most of it.

What remains remarkable is that some genius has found ways to make each piece of it uncomfortable, especially the beds. But should you be too sick or tired to care, they'll stick a few tubes in your arm and up your—hopefully only your nose—to make certain you appreciate modern health science.

Trained Personnel

The availability of doctors and nurses, with their supporting teams and equipment, are the primary reason that your hospital room costs more a night than the Plaza Hotel in New York City. There is an economic imperative that urges you to get out of that atmosphere the moment health conditions permit it.

Extended Care Places

People who are ready to leave the hospital, but are not able to go home, journey into a setting that combines group living and some level of medical supervision that is adequate to the need. The term *assisted living* may be used. The place may be called a hospital annex, a rest home, board and care, group home, or something like that. The cost is less. People who don't regain sufficient vitality for full independence often spend the rest of their lives in these places.

Infection

There is an old saw that says: If you weren't sick when you went into the hospital, the bugs you'll pick up while there will take care of the oversight. Extended care places have the same liability. No one wants infection to be so ever present, but it is.

The safest place for you to be sick is at home.

Home Care at Home

Even if you have insurance or a bankroll to cover the alarming cost of going somewhere else to be sick, home—someone's home—is where the health is. A loved one's home may be a workable idea. Your own home, perhaps with assistance that drops in every day, could be a better decision.

Help with Home Care

Professional Home Visitors

You will find that many of the companies that advertise visiting caregivers have mildly dementia-afflicted clients in mind or the merely feeble. When you tell them that you've got serious cancer, they beat a hasty retreat.

Your oncologist's team or your hospital should have highly qualified, trustworthy people to suggest. If not, contact:

- The American Cancer Society has great experience helping cancer patients find quality home care: 800-227-2345
- Medicare will provide you with a list of its certified home health care agencies: 800-633-4227
- For more on Medicare and Medicaid entitlements: 877-267-2323
- The Department of Veterans Affairs (VA) will cover home health care services for vets who are at least 50% disabled due to a service-related condition. If you are a Vietnam vet, myeloma is service related; call 800-827-1000

The National Association for Home Care (NAHC) publishes *How to Choose a Home Care Agency: A Consumer's Guide.* Call 202-547-7424 for a free copy. The NAHC also maintains a database of more than 20,000 prescreened home care and hospice agencies. Advisors at that phone number may also try to help you find the best way to fund the things you need.

Doctors and Nurses Make House Calls

Yes, there are both doctors and nurses making house calls. Discuss your needs with your primary care physician. The social worker attached to your hospital also knows about these professionals and how to hook you up with them.

Freelancers

People sometimes discover that home care availability has a time limit or a waiting period, or some other landmine buried in the fine print. There seems no alternative but to be creative. Lots of strategies are considered. Perhaps there is a teenager in the neighborhood who can help, or a housekeeper, or someone who may move in and trade health care for room and board.

Amateurs are a very dangerous option. People steal. People leave at just the wrong time. The horror stories abound. If circumstances force one of these alternatives on you, be wary.

Your Spouse

That line that was tossed off during your wedding vows about *for better or worse, in sickness and in health,* has now come home to roost. A spouse must do what he or she can. Many times, the spouse steps up, learns about daily care, and makes the necessary lifestyle and work changes. When that happens, the rewards are great.

Some spouses are unresponsive, and may even expect fulltime care equal to or greater than the patient's. This problem has to be faced and matter-of-factly dealt with. Seek counseling.

Emergency Care

Be certain that the help you need will be promptly at your door if you dial 911. If you live where rapid response paramedics aren't available, consider moving.

20

When Bad News Gets Worse: Don't Be Surprised

Jim Tamkin, MD

The hand that is dealt to a myeloma patient may seem unwinnable. Appearances can be deceiving. Don't give up.

Yes, it is possible—more than possible—for you to *also* have a heart attack, become diabetic, or contract some other serious health condition. Or maybe myeloma is your second, or third, serious health problem and you still have the others. As a patient being dealt these horrible cards, there are many concerns and questions. Albeit difficult and challenging, and even though you are afraid, these issues can often be successfully addressed.

Co-morbidity is the medical term given to this common situation. The impact of having two or more serious health conditions at once—on life expectancy and on treatment tolerance—is always considered when estimating the risks and benefits of various treatment plans. But complication does not rule out the possibility of victory. As Yogi Berra might say, it only complicates it.

Some of a myeloma patient's most likely additional medical conditions are:

- Kidney impairment: One in five myeloma patients experiences kidney failure. If the kidneys are not working properly, their ability to expel drugs in the urine may be less, leading to increased problems with toxicity (yellow skin, trouble sleeping, lack of energy, flu-like symptoms, feeling "puffy," noticeably reduced benefit or bad side effect from a drug). A change in drug treatment strategy is necessary.
- Anemia: Direct result of disease progression. Made worse by many myeloma drugs. Symptoms are fatigue, listlessness, pale appearance.
- Diabetes: Commonly used myeloma drugs can induce or exacerbate high blood sugar, leading to diabetes. This new co-morbidity is a risk that goes along with the benefit of a better, newer, but still imperfect process. *The diabetic condition that resulted does not mean that the treatment was a failure or a mistake.* If this raises a question or an alarm in your mind, please discuss it with your doctor immediately.
- Bone fractures: Myeloma begins in bones, causing them to weaken, leading to fractures.

Additional Co-Morbidities

The shock of learning that one has a deadly illness ought to raise awareness and heighten mental prowess. But in practice, the alarm wears off as one trudges through the endless cycles of diagnosis and treatment.

Impaired Cognition

Some of the mainstay treatments for myeloma, particularly extended bouts of chemotherapy, make concentration and recall more difficult. A patient can be aware of this and make every effort to counter it, and still experience loss. Mental acuity can come back later. Meanwhile, a caring helper who stays close, keeps records, and helps with daily chores such as pill taking is very valuable.

Depression

One-third of patients experience some sort of psychological distress, most often depression. Among the depressed, those who feel alone are the most likely victims. Financial worries and family discord are also common culprits.

Psychiatry, leaders in places of worship, family counseling, support groups, and other sources of effective help await those who are depressed. Seek the help of a qualified professional.

Weight Loss

Most of us will gain weight if we are not careful. So the idea of losing a few pounds may seem attractive. For myeloma patients, even a limited weight loss, less than 5%, can flag a possible co-morbidity. That is why your weight is regularly monitored by your medical team.

Drug Interactions

As we age, body fat increases, kidney function decreases, our livers get smaller, and blood flow decreases. The number of medications increases. These bring about an increased risk of potential problems. The therapeutics you're taking become far more critical. Regularly review the complete list with your medical team and your pharmacist to assess for potential drug interactions. All vitamins and herbs, including herb teas, *must be on this list.*

Poor Diet

If your diet does not include all the basic food groups (if you are a vegetarian, for instance), that is important information for your medical team, as well. This is not to criticize your diet, which may be exactly right for you. This is to help you make certain that your medical team does not make an assumption that is incorrect.

Co-Morbidities Pick on the Elderly

As we age, we're more apt to get sick. Our immune systems become less effective. Stamina goes down, too. Now myeloma enters the picture. Both the disease itself and the side effects of treating it open doors we try hard to keep closed. Along come these additional health issues, and conditions that are side effects of treatment and drugs. The situation, to put it mildly, ain't for sissies.

Does Advancing Age Reduce Treatment Options?

Infirmity can limit treatment options. But infirmity can occur at any age. Seniority alone has very little bearing on cancer treatment options. In particular, the stem cell and other transplant procedures that are important to many myeloma patients no longer have age limits. (Your health insurance provider may not know that.)

The Comprehensive Geriatric Assessment

Advancing age and the stresses of sickness will diminish the capacities of some. The Comprehensive Geriatric Assessment, a nationally recognized evaluation form, is increasingly used to measure it. A person's ability to maintain an independent life and to cope with the challenges of illness are obvious matters to be measured. This guide also helps predict complications and side effects of the life ahead of a myeloma patient.

Medicare and Insurance Company Conflicts

Both government-backed and private health insurers will struggle to understand the necessity for the drugs and treatments faced by myeloma patients. When co-morbidities are added, these folks can become confused and belligerent, as you have probably already observed.

In addition to heart attacks and other large issues, you may need treatment for cataracts, other eye conditions, dental problems, or hearing damage caused by the drugs you must take. Get your medical team to forecast all possible repercussions of proposed treatments. Get your public or private insurer to acknowledge them and to agree to provide the support you will need before beginning the treatment.

An Economic Co-Morbidity: Don’t Get Fired

If myeloma is a new condition, and if you are employed, involve your boss in your situation. You need your employer to be actively on your side, for lots of reasons.

To Be, or Not to Be (Sick); That Is a Question...

You have choices in dealing with all the tests, diagnoses, treatments, and the associated co-morbid and psychological issues. Three critical factors have to be kept in balance.

The first is the condition of your disease and its co-morbidities. There may be important reasons to take an aggressive pathway, even though it will have punishing side effects. Or it may be possible that a more comfortable treatment plan will bring you to the same or nearly same destination. If you belong to a myeloma support group, this is a useful matter to ask the group about. Perhaps there are friends there who have been down the paths you are considering. Your medical team may also have advice.

The second choice has to do with the preferences and capabilities of your medical team and the facilities it uses. There are growing numbers of myeloma treatment centers that use drug therapies for patients at most stages of this disease. Other hospitals, including three that are world famous for their success, prescribe stem cell transplants for most of their myeloma patients. You cannot know which treatment is most likely to be best for you. So whichever school of thought your medical team comes from, it is good to get a wholly independent second opinion.

The third factor that usually enters into the decision equation is time. You have an aggressive cancer and perhaps other health conditions that worry both you and your loved ones. You may feel that you need to do something quickly. And you may be right. But you need to understand that "watchful waiting" is also the right thing to do in certain circumstances. So, take the time you need to be certain that when you act, it is a thoughtful choice.

Patient-Centric Treatment

You, the patient, are usually the first to notice when you have a new health problem. Equally, you are the first to note (and often suffer from) its consequences. You are often the one who points the condition out to your doctor. Later, you have the first and often best sense of how the fix for what ails you is working.

We call all this *patient-centric treatment.* It is vital to the successful management of myeloma and becomes a doubly important strategy when co-morbidities are present.

Patient-centric treatment requires that you, the patient, become part of the medical team—as eyes and ears. Your careful, methodical, thorough analysis of how you feel and how treatment improved or failed to improve your health makes many parts of your medical team's effort more effective.

Do not—ever—go to a treatment or an examination and just sit there. Your team needs your thoughtful engagement. Equally, it needs your inquiry when you don't understand.

New Treatment Tools and Concepts Brighten the Picture

The newest, most effective treatments for myeloma discourage co-morbidities. Surgical procedures are less extensive. Lower doses of drugs are the new norm. The disease is beaten back more effectively. Organ function is less affected, and stronger, faster recovery is expected.

Additional Reading

As both a scientist and a patient, I shuttle back and forth between treatment centers and my medical journals. It is not a condition I recommend. You may even consider it a co-morbidity. Should you feel a need to be similarly burdened, a list of some of the reading I have found most informative follows.

Balducci, L, Extermann, M. Management of cancer in the older person: a practical approach. *Oncologist* 2000; 5:224.

Extermann, M, Aapro, M, Bernabei, R, et al. Use of comprehensive geriatric assessment in older cancer patients: recommendations from the task force on

CGA of the International Society of Geriatric Oncology (SIOG). *Crit Rev Oncol Hematol* 2005; 55:241.

Extermann, M, Overcash, J, Lyman, GH, et al. Comorbidity and functional status are independent in older cancer patients. *J Clin Oncol* 1998; 16:1582.

Gupta, SK, Lamont, EB. Patterns of presentation, diagnosis, and treatment in older patients with colon cancer and comorbid dementia. *J Am Geriatr Soc* 2004; 52:1681.

Hamerman, D. Toward an understanding of frailty. *Ann Intern Med* 1999; 130:945.

Hurria, A, Gupta, S, Zauderer, M, et al. Developing a cancer-specific geriatric assessment: a feasibility study. *Cancer* 2005; 104:1998.

Hurria, A, Leung, D, Trainor, K, et al. Factors influencing treatment patterns of breast cancer patients age 75 and older. *Crit Rev Oncol Hematol* 2003; 46:121.

Hutchins, LF, Unger, JM, Crowley, JJ, et al. Underrepresentation of patients 65 years of age or older in cancer-treatment trials. *N Engl J Med* 1999; 341:2061.

Ingram, SS, Seo, PH, Martell, RE, et al. Comprehensive assessment of the elderly cancer patient: the feasibility of self-report methodology. *J Clin Oncol* 2002; 20:770.

Kua, J. The prevalence of psychological and psychiatric sequelae of cancer in the elderly—how much do we know? *Ann Acad Med Singapore* 2005; 34:250.

Langa, KM, Valenstein, MA, Fendrick, AM, et al. Extent and cost of informal caregiving for older Americans with symptoms of depression. *Am J Psychiatry* 2004; 161:857.

Newcomb, PA, Carbone, PP. Cancer treatment and age: patient perspectives. *J Natl Cancer Inst* 1993; 85:1580.

Overcash, JA, Beckstead, J, Extermann, M, Cobb, S. The abbreviated comprehensive geriatric assessment (aCGA): a retrospective analysis. *Crit Rev Oncol Hematol* 2005; 54:129.

Rao, AV, Hsieh, F, Feussner, JR, Cohen, HJ. Geriatric evaluation and management units in the care of the frail elderly cancer patient. *J Gerontol Biol Sci Med Sci* 2005; 60:798.

Repetto, L, Fratino, L, Audisio, RA, et al. Comprehensive geriatric assessment adds information to Eastern Cooperative Oncology Group performance status in elderly cancer patients: an Italian Group for Geriatric Oncology Study. *J Clin Oncol* 2002; 20:494.

Stafford, RS, Cyr, PL. The impact of cancer on the physical function of the elderly and their utilization of health care. *Cancer* 1997; 80:1973.

Trimble, EL, Carter, CL, Cain, D, et al. Representation of older patients in cancer treatment trials. *Cancer* 1994; 74:2208.

Tucci, A, Ferrari, S, Bottelli, C, et al. A comprehensive geriatric assessment is more effective than clinical judgment to identify elderly diffuse large cell lymphoma patients who benefit from aggressive therapy. *Cancer* 2009; 115:4547.

Epiloge

Pat Killingsworth

Don't believe the stats.

Being diagnosed with multiple myeloma changes your life forever. There are countless reasons to bemoan your new normal; a world of blood draws, tests, and chemotherapy—and possibly a stem cell transplant down the road.

But for many, living with multiple myeloma isn't all bad. Many survivors continue to work and grow. You make new friends. You discover that you are capable of overcoming things you never dreamed you could. And if you navigate all of this just right, you may end up a stronger, better person for it.

Contributors to this book have intentionally avoided survival statistics. There are a number of reasons. These statistics lump everyone together—patients with serious pre-existing conditions, older patients, patients who are diagnosed late, difficult-to-treat high-risk patients—which skews the numbers, making them highly misleading.

Here's some good news: Myeloma research has been so successful that overall survival data are often outdated before it's even recorded.

Try and remember that you are not a statistic. So whether your doctor tells you that the average patient lives five years or a decade doesn't matter. You aren't *average,* are you?

If this book has taught you anything, it's that becoming an informed multiple myeloma patient can help you live a longer, better life. So don't let reading things like *There is no cure for multiple myeloma* discourage you from continuing your myeloma education. I'm constantly amazed at how many positive experiences I have gleaned from what could be viewed as a negative prognosis.

My new calling as a myeloma activist and medical writer has granted me access to the best and brightest minds focused on multiple myeloma. You (the reader) have just finished a gift from well over a hundred patients, caregivers, their health care teams, researchers, drug developers, myeloma nonprofits, government agencies, bankers, lawyers, CPAs, and numerous others impacted by the disease. TBA. Their Best Advice. The foundation behind this book.

But learning from and experiencing the energy of these dedicated, hardworking men and women isn't the best part of my job. No, it's meeting my fellow patients and caregivers. People like you and me, working hard every day to overcome obstacles that none of us dreamed we would ever face a short time ago.

If I hadn't been diagnosed with multiple myeloma, I never would have had a chance to meet Don Wright, a 70-year-old who has run marathons in all 50 states since his diagnosis in 2003. Or Jim Bond, a 21-year survivor who calmed me down in a Boston men's room, when my bone and muscle pain was so bad I wasn't sure I wanted to live.

I have been exchanging e-mails with Ed Wolfman, a fellow myeloma survivor in California, for years. Ed and I graduated from the University of Wisconsin about the same time. We didn't know each other back then. But it turns out that Ed knew one of this book's authors, Dr. Jim Tamkin.

Here is what Ed had to say about Jim: "When I was first diagnosed, it was suggested that I speak with Dr. Tamkin. I did. We had breakfast together (he paid!). I was frightened and completely uninformed of what was ahead of me. Dr. Tamkin laid out the important aspects of dealing with the disease. He was a virile, positive man who gave me a huge boost into thinking that things would work out."

Ed was diagnosed more than seven years ago and is doing great! A father and loving husband, Ed is working, traveling, and living what most would consider a normal, fulfilling life.

Keeping Ed's words in mind, I decided to ask a number of longtime myeloma survivors for their secrets to living with this disease and would like to share a few of those with you.

Let's start in Florida, where 15-year survivor Roz Jarrett lives. Roz remains in full remission after undergoing an autologous (her own cells) stem cell transplant 14 years ago. Roz is a great-grandmother. She attributes her happy, healthy life to staying active and eating well. No matter how busy she gets, Roz walks every day. "Keep moving!," Roz tells anyone who asks. (Are you listening?)

Elliot Recht, from San Diego, California, is also a 15-year survivor. Elliot is still working, and founded a large myeloma support group there. He wishes that he had paid more attention to the mental health part of his cancer. His suggestion: "Eliminate the people, places and things that cause aggravation in your life." I'll second that advice.

So, you think 15 years is impressive? Patricia Harwood, Minneapolis, was diagnosed early in 1996 and underwent an allogeneic (donor) stem cell transplant later that same year. Although Pat has since relapsed, her doctor at Mayo Clinic is using a combination of drugs to keep her myeloma under control. Pat's advice for newly diagnosed patients: *Don't look at the stats. You have a future!* Pat also wanted me to remind patients and caregivers that your treatment is toxic, and that's what's making you sick. Once your myeloma is in check, you can move on and begin to lead a quality life again.

Californian Mary Ann Ming-Mosley is an amazing woman—and a 20-year multiple myeloma survivor.

Diagnosed in 1992, Mary Ann underwent her first of two autologous stem cell transplants in 1994. Mary Ann is a strikingly beautiful African American woman with a dark, glowing complexion and a sparkle in her eye. When you engage her, you instantly sense Mary Ann's love for life and you feel an indescribable energy.

I have met Mary Ann a number of times. When I called to interview her for this book, she had just returned from her local cancer center after undergoing an infusion of a newly FDA-approved drug, Kyprolis. As you can guess, Mary Ann has experienced every possible therapy over the past 20 years. Fortunately, most of them have worked; sometimes only for a year or two, but nimble, out-of-the-box thinking is what keeps us going.

Mary Ann shared a number of tips for newly diagnosed patients: "Become your own best advocate, join a myeloma support group and use the resources provided by the International Myeloma Foundation." But to me, it isn't what Mary Ann says that's important. It's what she's done and how she's done it.

Mary Ann's spirituality also shines through. By placing faith in a higher power, Mary Ann has been able to focus on her recovery.

These brave men and women are my heroes. Knowing them has given me hope. Hope that, like them, I can persevere and live a long, productive life.

I believe that all long-lived multiple myeloma patients—those of us who defy the so-called odds—have one important thing in common: a deeply burning will to live.

As I came to grips with my unfortunate diagnosis, I began to focus on helping other multiple myeloma patients and caregivers as a way to rationalize my new lot in life. Like many others, mistakes were made, by both me and members of my health care team. I began to realize that, as Mary Ann suggests, I should become my own best advocate.

Knowledge is power, and I vowed I would learn as much as I can about myeloma therapy and how to live a longer and better life with my cancer. This calling—to help others do the same—has filled me with the deeply burning will to live.

There is no proof that being positive will help you live longer. Cancer is a powerful enemy. But staying positive and optimistic will improve your quality of life. That is probably the most important thing that all of those who have beaten the odds and outlived expectations have in common.

Dr. Tamkin opened this book very simply, *Hang in and hold on.* Jim did just that, dedicating his life to helping other myeloma patients and caregivers.

Take time to mourn your diagnosis. You have been dealt a rotten hand. But don't wallow and don't give up! Be hopeful, don't be afraid to ask for help, and don't forget that you aren't alone.

Glossary

Alkylating agent: A class of chemotherapy drugs that fight myeloma by blocking cancer cell division. Alkeran (melphalan) and Cytoxan (cyclophosphamide) are well-known compounds of this sort.

Allogeneic: Bone marrow or stem cells transplanted from another person are called *allogeneic.* For more, see *Transplantation.*

Anemia: Too few red blood cells. Normal hemoglobin score for women is between 11.7 and 16 on *CBC* tests; for men, normal score is between 12.4 and 15. Myeloma in bone marrow may block red blood cell production. Anemia causes shortness of breath, weakness, and fatigue, and can be very serious.

Anesthesia: Loss of feeling or awareness. Local anesthesia causes loss of feeling in a part of the body. General anesthesia puts a person to sleep.

Angiogenesis: Blood vessel formation, which usually accompanies the growth of malignant (cancerous) tissue.

Angiogenesis inhibitors: Drugs that cut off blood supply to tumors.

Antibody: A protein that white cells produce to fight a bacteria, virus, or tumor. Antibodies are now being manufactured to treat certain types of cancer.

Elotuzumab is an antibody being produced to fight multiple myeloma.

Antigen: A protein from a bacteria, virus, or tumor that causes the body to create antibodies.

Apheresis: Procedure in which blood is taken out of a vein and run into a machine that harvests one or more of its components. The remaining blood goes back to the patient. *Stem cells* are usually obtained in this way.

Apoptosis: Programmed cell death. The natural biochemical events that lead to the ending of the life of a cell. (Wikipedia: Between 50 and 70 billion cells die each day due to apoptosis in the average human adult.)

Autologous: In transplant therapy, *autologous* means that the patient is his or her own donor. For more, see *Transplantation.*

Benign: Doing little or no harm. Not cancerous.

Biopsy: The removal of a sample for lab study. Also called a pathological evaluation.

Bisphosphonate: A type of drug used to stop bones from dissolving. Aredia (pamidronate disodium) and Zometa (zoledronic acid) are best known.

Blood cells: Minute structures produced in the bone marrow, circulated in a liquid medium called blood plasma. There are three basic types: red, white, and platelets. (Stem cells, also in the blood, are baby white cells, available to become almost any sort of cell the body needs. See *Stem cells.)*

Blood count: The number of red blood cells, white blood cells, and platelets in a sample of blood. A complete blood count *(CBC)* also lists other things in the blood and measures a complex set of blood conditions.

Bone marrow: The soft, spongy tissue in the center of many bones that produces blood cells.

Bone marrow aspiration: The use of a needle to remove a sample of fluid and cells from the bone marrow for laboratory examination.

Bone marrow biopsy: The removal of a small amount of bone marrow, often from a hip bone; the study of the sample in a lab; and a report of findings.

Bone scan: A bone picture that can spot cancer. Bone scans can also show that drug therapy is working and that damaged bony areas are healing.

Brachytherapy: Radiation therapy. A radioactive material is placed inside or next to the area requiring treatment.

BUN (blood urea nitrogen): A laboratory test to evaluate kidney function by measuring the urea level in the blood. Diseases such as myeloma, which compromise kidney function, frequently lead to increased levels of BUN.

Calcium: A mineral found in bone. Elevated levels of calcium may be found in blood when bone destruction has taken place.

Cancer: A term for diseases in which abnormal (malignant) cells divide without control. Myeloma cancer cells can invade nearby tissues and spread through the bloodstream and lymph node systems.

Carcinogen: Any substance or agent that is directly involved in causing cancer.

CAT or CT scan, more formally called **computed (axial) tomography scan:** A test using computerized x-rays to create three-dimensional images of organs and structures inside the body. Often used to detect small areas of bone damage or soft tissue involvement. This type of machine has revolutionized the diagnosis of cancer and other diseases.

Catheter: A thin, flexible tube that may be inserted into any opening of the body. It is inserted into a vein in order to send in drugs, blood or nutrients. Catheters are also used in minimally invasive surgery, to take blood or to empty the bladder.

CBC: A complete blood count test uses a drawn sample to measure amounts of white blood cells, red blood cells, platelets, and other components of the blood.

Chemotherapy: The treatment of cancer with chemicals (drugs) designed to kill cancer cells or stop them from multiplying.

Chromosome: The fundamental strands of genetic material (DNA) that carry all of our genes. Normally, human cells contain 46 chromosomes. Tumor cells sometimes have more or fewer than 46 chromosomes.

Chronic: Persisting over a long period of time. Chronic does not imply incurable or fatal.

Clinical trial: The procedures by which new cancer treatments are tested in people. Clinical trials are conducted after experiments in animals and preliminary studies have shown that a new treatment method might be effective. Each study is designed to find better ways to prevent, detect, diagnose, or treat cancer and to answer scientific questions.

Colony-stimulating factors: A class of drugs that encourage bone marrow stem cells to divide and develop into white blood cells, platelets, and red blood cells. A process also called *mobilization.*

Creatinine: A compound normally excreted by kidneys. If kidneys are damaged, the amount of creatinine builds up, resulting in less efficient bodily waste management. The *serum creatinine test* is used to measure kidney function.

Diagnosis: The process of identifying a disease by its signs and symptoms.

Dialysis: A process that cleans a patient's blood by passing it through a machine that artificially replaces kidney function. Special filters may be used for myeloma patients.

DNA (deoxyribonucleic acid): The building block of our genetic material responsible for passing on hereditary characteristics and information on cell growth, division, and function.

Drug resistance: The development of resistance in cancer cells to a specific drug or drugs. If resistance develops, a patient in remission may relapse despite continued administration of anticancer drugs.

Edema: An abnormal accumulation of fluid or swelling within body tissues.

Efficacy: The ability of a drug to produce the desired therapeutic effect.

Electrophoresis: A lab test in which a blood plasma sample is exposed to an electric field that separates the proteins it contains into different classes. Reveals very important things about how myeloma has affected the patient's blood.

Gene: A biological unit of DNA capable of transmitting a single characteristic from parent to offspring. Genes are found in all cells in the body. When genes are missing or damaged, cancer may occur.

Genetic: Inherited; having to do with information that is passed from generation to generation through DNA in the genes.

Graft-versus-host disease (GVHD): Complication of *allogeneic transplants* resulting from donor immune cells recognizing the recipient's cells as foreign and mounting an attack against them. This is a serious problem. Drugs are available to combat it. Note: In some cases, a GVH reaction actually helps control the cancer.

Hematocrit (Hct): The percentage of red blood cells in the blood. A low hematocrit measurement indicates anemia. Normal *CBC* test levels for adult males range from 42 to 49; for adult females, 38 to 46. These values may vary slightly among different laboratories.

Hematologist: A doctor who specializes in diseases of the blood and bone marrow.

Hemoglobin: A substance found within red blood cells that carries oxygen from the lungs to the tissues in the body. Low hemoglobin levels are an indicator of *anemia.* The normal *CBC* test value in men is from 12.4 to 15g; in women, from 12.5 to 14g.

Hypercalcemia: A higher-than-normal level of calcium in the blood. This condition can cause a number of symptoms including loss of appetite, nausea, thirst, fatigue, muscle weakness, restlessness, and confusion. Because calcium can be toxic to the kidneys and heart, hypercalcemia is usually treated on an emergency basis.

Immunoglobulin: Any of a family of *antibodies* in the blood that fight infection.

Immunosuppression: Weakening of the immune system that causes a lowered ability to fight infection and disease. Immunosuppression often results from chemotherapy for the treatment of cancers. Note: Immunosuppression is sometimes deliberate, as when a patient is being prepared for transplant.

Indolent: Myeloma that is not aggressive. Not progressing.

Induction therapy: The initial treatment used to achieve remission in a newly diagnosed cancer patient.

Infusion: Administration of fluids or medications by intravenous injection (IV) into the bloodstream over a period of time.

Injection: Pushing a medication into the body with the use of a syringe and needle.

Lesion: Any area of abnormal tissue. A term used to describe a cut, an injury, an infected area, or a tumor. In myeloma, lesion can also refer to a *plasmacytoma;* a hole in the bone.

Lytic lesions: The damaged area of a bone where healthy bone has been eaten away.

M proteins (M spike): Abnormal *antibodies* (or *immunoglobulin)* found in the blood or urine of multiple myeloma patients. M protein levels are used to estimate the extent of myeloma disease and to determine the effectiveness of treatments. *M spike* refers to the sharp pattern shown by *electrophoresis* when an M protein is present.

Maintenance therapy: Treatment that is given to patients in remission to delay or prevent a relapse.

Malignant: Another word for cancerous. Describes a tendency to invade nearby tissue and spread to other parts of the body.

Metastasis: The spread of cancer from one part of the body to another by way of the lymph system or bloodstream.

MGUS (*m* onoclonal *g* ammopathy of *u* ndetermined *s* ignificance):

A condition without symptoms in which the *Mprotein* is present in blood or urine but there is no disease. All myeloma patients develop MGUS first, but only a few percent of the MGUS cases progress to myeloma.

Mobilization: Administration of *colony-stimulating factor* or *chemotherapy* to help move *stem cells* from the *bone marrow* into the blood-stream. This increases the number of stem cells that can be collected for a stem cell transplant. See also *Transplantation.*

Monoclonal antibodies: Manufactured compounds designed to find and lock a marker onto cancer cells for diagnostic or treatment purposes. They can be used alone, or they can be used to deliver other drugs, toxins, or radioactive material to tumor cells.

MRI (magnetic resonance imaging): A diagnostic test that uses magnetic energy and radio waves, rather than x-rays, to produce detailed two- or three-dimensional images of organs and structures inside the body. Gives very fine resolution of soft tissues, notably encroachments on the spinal cord, but is less accurate for bone lesions.

Neoplasm: Any new growth of tissue or cells. May be *benign* or *malignant.*

Neuropathy: Disorder of the nerves that can result in numbness, burning, or tingling. When the hands or feet are affected, it is referred to as "peripheral" neuropathy.

Neutropenia: Too few neutrophils in the blood. This is often a side effect of chemotherapy. Neutropenia can be prevented or treated with a synthetic hormone called G-CSF, contained in Neulasta (pegfilgrastim) and Neupogen (filgrastim).

Neutrophil: A type of white blood cell essential to fighting infection.

Oncologist: A doctor who specializes in treating cancer.

Osteonecrosis of the jaw: A previously rare jaw problem now being observed in some myeloma patients taking *bisphosphonates.* The condition produces bone damage around the tooth sockets in the jaws and bone necrosis or loss of bone that can lead to loose or lost teeth, sharp edges of exposed bone, bone spurs, and the breaking loose of small particles of dead bone. Symptoms may not be obvious at first, and may include pain, swelling, numbness, a heavy jaw feeling, or loosening of a tooth.

Palliative: Treatment intended to improve feelings of well-being, to relieve symptoms, or to control the growth of myeloma—but not to cure.

Pathology: The study of disease through the examination of tissues, organs, and body fluids. A doctor who does this is called a pathologist.

PET (positron emission tomography) scan: A diagnostic test that uses a sophisticated camera and computer to detect areas of cells that are living and growing more rapidly than others. It may find areas of cancer by detecting their growth, rather than the space they occupy, as in CT and MRI scans. PET scans have become vital for myeloma staging and assessment.

Placebo: An inactive substance or treatment sometimes used in clinical trials for comparison with an experimental drug. A placebo has no beneficial effect.

Plasma: The part of the blood in which red blood cells, white blood cells, and platelets are suspended.

Plasma cell: A type of white blood cell found in bone marrow that normally produces antibodies to fight infection. This is the cell that becomes cancerous in myeloma patients.

As cancerous plasma cells go about the business of causing bone, organ, other tissue, and nerve damage within the body, an *M protein* is produced. Its level, the *M spike,* is an indicator of response to therapy or of worsening disease.

Plasmacytoma: A single tumor or collection of cancerous plasma cells in a single location.

Platelets (thrombocytes): One of the three kinds of circulating blood cells (others being the red blood cells and white blood cells). Platelets are the major defense against bleeding, as they plug up breaks in the blood vessel walls and stimulate blood clot formation. A normal *CBC* platelet count is 150,000 to 300,000.

Port implanted: A small, quarter-sized disc with a soft center that is surgically placed just below the skin in the chest or abdomen. A tube (catheter) from it goes into a large vein or artery. Fluids, drugs or blood products can be infused through it and blood can be drawn from it.

Prognosis: A statement about the likely outcome or course of a medical condition, the chance of recovery, or the life expectancy. A patient's prognosis is based on signs, symptoms, circumstances, and clinical findings, largely influenced by statistics and the experience of the physician who provides the assessment.

Progression-free survival: The time period during which the patient survives and the cancer does not become worse.

Progressive disease: Disease that is becoming worse, as documented by tests. In most cases, relapsed and refractory disease can be considered progressive.

Proteasome: A complex of enzymes found within cells. Proteasomes play a key role in the regulation of cell function and growth by breaking down and clearing out proteins after they've done their job and are no longer needed. Some cancer cells also depend on proteasomes to grow.

Protocol: A precisely written description of a treatment regimen; the patient's instruction when participating in a clinical trial or research program.

Radiation therapy: Treatment with x-rays, gamma rays, or electrons to damage or kill cells. The radiation may come from outside the body (external radiation), or from radioactive materials placed inside the body near the tumor (implant radiation, also called *brachytherapy).*

Radiologist: A doctor who specializes in creating and interpreting images of areas inside the body through the use of x-rays and other imaging techniques (such as ultrasound, MRI, and radioactive tracers) to diagnose and investigate disease.

Recurrence: The return of disease that had disappeared. In myeloma cases, recurrence is also known as *refractory* myeloma. The disease that comes back may not respond to drugs in the old way and may cause new problems for the patient.

Red blood cells (erythrocytes): Cells in the blood that contain hemoglobin and deliver oxygen to and take carbon dioxide from the body.

Refractory: Disease that has become unresponsive to the treatment being given.

Regression: The shrinkage of cancer growth, usually as the result of therapy. In a complete regression, all tumors disappear; in a partial regression, some tumor remains.

Relapse: Disease that initially responded to therapy but then begins to progress again.

Remission: Complete or partial disappearance of the signs and symptoms of cancer, usually occurring as the result of therapy.

- **Complete remission (CR):** CR is the absence of *M protein* from blood and urine; absence of myeloma cells from the *bone marrow* and other areas of myeloma involvement; clinical remission and the improvement of other laboratory parameters to normal. CR is not the same thing as cure.
- **Partial remission (PR):** PR is a reduced level of disease, though some is still detected. Some treatment centers consider more than 50% reduction in myeloma cells—but less than 75%—to be partial remission. Other clinicians call anything greater than 50% reduction in disease a partial remission.

Serum creatinine test: Measures kidney function. See *Creatinine.*

Side effects: Problems caused by drugs and radiation. Common side effects of myeloma treatment are fatigue, nausea, vomiting, decreased blood cell counts, hair loss, radiation burns, and mouth sores. Severe infections can also begin in the mouth and cataracts may develop.

Stable disease: When myeloma has not responded to therapy for a time, nor progressed, it falls into this category. When the disease has partially responded to therapy and since then remained stable, it may be put in this category. Synonym for *progression-free survival.* With slow-moving myeloma, stabilization can now last for many years.

Staging: An organized process of exams and tests to determine the extent of cancer in the body.

Stem cells: Immature white blood cells used as building and rebuilding blocks in many places in the body. Normal stem cells give rise to normal blood components, including red cells, white cells and platelets. Stem cells are primarily located in the bone marrow, but are also found in peripheral (circulating) blood, and can be harvested for *transplantation.*

Steroid: A class of fat-soluble chemicals—including cortisone, male and female sex hormones—that are often given to myeloma patients, along with one or more anticancer drugs, to help control the myeloma and to reduce damaging effects of the disease on the body.

Supportive care: Treatment given to prevent, control, or relieve symptoms, complications, and side effects and to improve the patient's comfort and quality of life.

Systemic therapy: Treatment using substances that travel through the bloodstream, reaching and affecting cancer cells throughout the body.

Transfusion: The transfer of blood or blood products.

Transplantation: *Stem cells* are used to restart the body's blood-forming process after high-dose *chemotherapy* and sometimes radiation have wiped out both the myeloma and the patient's good white cells. *Transplantation* is not a treatment. It's the repair job that follows treatment.

- **Bone marrow transplantation:** The process of collecting *bone marrow* and infusing it into a patient. This procedure is used less frequently today than it was.
- **Peripheral blood stem cell transplantation:** Healthy *stem cells* from a patient's circulating blood system (not from the bone marrow) are removed and stored before the patient receives high-dose *chemotherapy* and possibly radiation therapy to destroy the cancer cells. The *stem cells* are then returned to the patient, where they can repopulate

the bone marrow and then produce new blood cells to replace cells destroyed by the chemo.

- **Allogeneic:** The infusion of *bone marrow* or *stem cells* from one individual (donor) to another (recipient). A patient receives *bone marrow* or *stem cells* from a compatible, though not genetically identical, donor.
- **Autologous:** A procedure in which *stem cells* are removed from a patient's own blood and then are given back to the patient following intensive treatment.
- **Syngeneic:** The infusion of *bone marrow* or *stem cells* from one identical twin into another.

Tumor: An abnormal mass of tissue that results from excessive cell division. It may either be *benign* or *malignant.*

Tumor marker: A substance in blood or other body fluids providing evidence that a person has cancer. May also help target cancer cells.

Vaccine: A substance prepared from the causative agent of a disease, its products, or a synthetic substitute. Administered to produce or artificially increase immunity.

Waldenstrom's macroglobulemia: A rare type oflymphoma. Not myeloma.

White blood cells (leukocytes): General term for a variety of cells that develop in the bone marrow and are responsible for the body's immune defenses. Specific white blood cells include basophils, eosinophils, lymphocytes, monocytes, and neutrophils. A normal *CBC* count is 5,000 to 10,000 and may be elevated or depressed by a wide variety of conditions. *Chemotherapy* usually causes low counts.

X-ray: High-energy ionizing radiation used in low doses to study myeloma and in high doses to treat it.

Acknowledgments

When Jim Tamkin and I began this process, it was immediately apparent that the work of sorting through and assembling the best advice of leading multiple myeloma voices from all over the country would take years and cost an alarming amount of money. "The book" wasn't a book. It was a nonprofit foundation, governed by State of California and federal tax agencies, selflessly supported by several hundred professionals and patients, anchored by a website, requiring a literary agent, a law firm, a publisher, bankers, a board of directors, employees, overhead, equipment ... plus the manuscript, which now stands at something north of 65,000 words, and is in its umpteenth iteration.

The foundation has received both financial and material help from others in the four years that have followed. Among them:

Anita Chambers
Celgene Corporation
Malin and Lenore Dollinger
Dorsey and Whitney: Ulrika Vettleson, Claire Topp, and Greg Tamkin
Genentech
Azhar Hameed
Dawna Houston
International Myeloma Foundation
Pat Killingsworth

John and Kathleen Killip
Soterios F. Menzelos
Millennium: The Takeda Oncology Company
Multiple Myeloma Research Foundation
Onyx Pharmaceuticals, an Amgen subsiderary
Jim and Fern Tamkin
Vasek and Anna Maria Polak Charitable Foundation
Karen Visel
Wells Fargo Bank Foundation
Writers House: Al Zuckerman

On behalf of Malin Dollinger, MD, TBA Foundation Chairman, and in memory of our friend, Jim Tamkin, MD, it is my honor to acknowledge these generosities.

Sincerely,
Dave Visel

Notes

Introduction

Treatment and research in 2012: A calculation based on the 2012 findings of the Surveillance, Epidemiology, and End Results (SEER) Program of the National Cancer Institute. seer.cancer.gov

A usually harmless condition: See the watershed study, "Monoclonal Gammopathy of Undetermined Significance," by Robert A. Kyle, MD, *The American Journal of Medicine* 06/1978; 64(5):814-826.

How either disease selects: Burton Dickey, MD, Professor and Chair, Department of Pulmonary Medicine Cardiopulmonary Center, MD Anderson Cancer Center, Houston, TX, himself a myeloma patient, points out that a defective DNA replication process leads to these diseases. Interview with Dave Visel.

Chapter 1

Research indicates: A. Waxman et al., "Racial Disparities in Incidence and Outcome in Multiple Myeloma: A Population-Based Study," *Blood* (American Society of Hematology), September 7, 2010; doi:10.1182/blood-2010-07-298760; *Cancer Facts &*

Figures for African Americans 2009-2010, published by the American Cancer Society and available for download at its website, www.cancer.org

At this point in her essay: "Let Real Healthcare Reform Begin with Me, "by Valerie Ulene, MD, *Los Angeles Times* [essay], April 13, 2009.

Chapter 2

"Your perspective is different": This section is based on a taped interview done in 2009 with Dave Visel.

Green tea and Velcade: Millennium Pharmaceuticals.

Iron supplements and Aredia or Zometa: Integrative Medicine Service, Memorial Sloan-Kettering Cancer Center.

More than 1,200 scientific studies: From an interview with Dave Visel, Torrance, California, March 5, 2004. First appeared in *Living with Cancer,* by Dave Visel (Rutgers University Press, 2006).

Chapter 3

At some point during the experience: "Secret Shame," by Don Vaughan, *Cure Magazine,* Winter 2011.

Chapter 5

Cognoscenti began the practice: Origins, by Eric Partridge (New York: Macmillan, 1958): 109.

One in five myeloma patients: 20% to 60% of patients will present with some degree of renal (kidney) insufficiency or renal failure throughout their disease, not just at diagnosis, but throughout. Beth Faiman, RN, MSN, APRN-BC, AOCN, Multiple Myeloma Program, Cleveland Clinic Foundation, Oncology Nursing Society Meeting, March 16, 2011.

A nutritionist will work with you: David Allen August, MD, et al., A.S.P.E.N. "Clinical Guidelines: Nutritional Support Therapy During Adult Anticancer Treatment," *Journal of Parenteral and Enteral Nutrition* 33, no.5 (September/October 2009): 472–500.

Chapter 6

How to Fix Medicare and Medicaid Disputes: MAXIMUS Federal Services.

The Agent Orange (and Other Herbicides) Special Circumstance: For more, see www.publichealth.va.gov/exposures/agentorange/vietnam.asp and thomas.loc.gov/cgi-bin/bdquery/z?d102:HR00556:@@@L&summ2=m&

If you served in the Navy offshore: See www.bluewaternavy.org/NHL/nhl.htm; www.bluewaternavy.org/Thailand/thaibase.htm

Those stationed near the Korean Demilitarized Zone: www.publichealth.va.gov/exposures/agentorange/korea.asp

If you were stationed at Fort Detrick: www.publichealth.va.gov/docs/agentorange/reviews/ao_newsletter_jul01.pdf

Everybody else who served: Ibid.

The Radiation Exposure Compensation Act: www.justice.gov/civil/common/reca.html

Atomic veterans: www.publichealth.va.gov/exposures/radiation/radiation-risk-activity.asp

Investigate "Medical Tourism": "Surgical Tourism," by Chad Terhune, *Los Angeles Times,* November 17, 2012; and "Competitive Care," by Margherita Stancati, *Wall Street Journal,* April 13, 2010. Also see health-tourism.com

Chapter 10

In 1959, it was discovered: C. Jones, *R.I.P.: The Complete Book of Death and Dying* (HarperCollins, 1997): 35.

Chapter 11

This and other names: Organic Chemistry, Structure and Function, by Vollhardt and Schore, "Rules for Naming Organic Molecules," W.H. Freeman; 5th edition pp.71–76.

"The biopharmaceutical industry's scientists…": "Will Washington Find the Cure for Cancer?" Kenneth C. Frazier, *Wall Street Journal,* July 12, 2011.

According to a current study: Go to eHealthMe.com (listcompiled in 2012).

Families of Drugs: Based on categories and classifications reported by www.cancercare.org

The first mention of a paid experimental: John P. Bull, "The Historical Development of Clinical Therapeutic Trials," *Journal of Chronic Diseases* 10, no.3 (1959): 219.

Drugs and Their Potential Side Effects: Information in this section is from manufacturer websites and "Managing Side Effects of Novel Agents," a lecture by Beth Faiman, NP, Cleveland Clinic, sponsored by the International Myeloma Foundation, March 3, 2011. Additional sources for specific drugs are provided in individual notes following.

Decadron (dexameth asone): Possible side effects when used as part of a chemotherapy protocol, Cleveland Clinic Foundation, 2005.

Deltasone (prednisone): MedicineNet, Inc.

Elotuzumab: Philippe Moreau, M, University Hospital, Nantes, France. Findings at the 47th Annual Meeting of the American Society of Clinical Oncology (ASCO), June 4–8, 2011.

Kyprolis (carfilzomib): Onyx Pharmaceuticals.

Thrombocytopenia (low platelet count) vitamin therapy: Recommendations compiled by Beth Faiman, NP, Cleveland Clinic, in a Cleveland Clinic pamphlet for myeloma patients.

"Chemical compounds in chocolate": Direct quotes in this section are from Melissa Gaskill, "Sweet Relief: Could Chocolate Prevent Cancer?" *Cure* (Summer 2012).

Chapter 12

It's a side effect of your condition: Updates from ASCO, poster sessions of Jesus San Miguel, M, and colleagues, June 6, 2011.

Don't be surprised if your ability to concentrate: "The Fog That Follows Chemotherapy," Jane E. Brody, *Personal Health,* August 3, 2009.

Chemo May Open the Door to Infection: "Fighting Back, Neutropenia Means Losing Protection from Infection," Lindsay Ray, *Cure Magazine,* March 2, 2011.

Current thinking among scientists: M. Chesi, E. Nardini, L.A. Brents, et al.," Frequent translocation (4;14)(p16.3;q32.3) in multiple myeloma is associated with increased expression and activating mutations of fibroblast growth factor receptor 3," *Nature Genetics* 16, no.3 (1997): 260–264; www.ncbi.nlm.gov/pubmed/92077913/21/12

The American Ophthalmological Society advises: See the American Ophthalmological Society website, www.aosonline.org

Chapter 13

Today, about 70%: "Radiation Therapy, Vertebroplasty, and Kyphoplasty: Three Treatments for Myeloma Bone Disease," Amrita Purohit, *The Myeloma Beacon,* January 23, 2009.

Helical Tomotherapy: Information in this section is from the City of Hope website, www.cityofhope.org

Chapter 14

All myeloma patients will need to undergo: Thank you to Pat Killingsworth for much of the information in this section.

Skeletal Complications: Details for this section provided by the Institute for Myeloma and Bone Cancer Research, www.imbcr.org.

According to a recent study by James Berenson, MD: Melissa Cobleigh, "Researchers Identify Factors Associated with Improved Survival in Myeloma Patients after Surgery for Skeletal Complications," *The Myeloma Beacon,* November 3, 2010.

Chapter 15

Bone marrow produces: American Society of Clinical Oncologists (ASCO), www.asco.org

The nation's leading myeloma treatment centers: *Multidisciplinary Team Approach: Managing the Newly Diagnosed Patient,* by Sergio A. Giralt, MD; Donald HarveyIII, PharmD; Beth Faiman, NP; Managing Myeloma, MediCom Worldwide, Inc., 101 Washington Street, Morrisville, PA 19067, 215-337-9991, July 18, 2012.

"I think we are all very gratified": "When Is Stem Cell Transplantation Indicated for the Treatment of Multiple

Myeloma?," by Ann F. Mohrbacher, MD, Assistant Professor of Medicine, Division of Hematology, University of Southern California, Managing Myeloma©2009 MediCom Worldwide, Inc.

Medics are inclined to go: Multidisciplinary Team Approach: Managing the Newly Diagnosed Patient, by Sergio A. Giralt, MD; Donald Harvey III, PharmD; Beth Faiman, NP; Managing Myeloma, MediCom Worldwide, Inc., 101 Washington Street, Morrisville, PA 19067, 215-337-9991, July 18, 2012.

Dr. Mak initiated a chemo-based plan: For seminal thinking behind this treatment strategy, see *Journal of Hematotherapy & Stem Cell Research* 11, no.1 (February 2002): 33–47; doi:10.1089/152581602753448522

The words remission, relapse, and refractory disease: MyMultipleMyeloma.com, a service to myeloma patients and their caregivers provided by Millennium Pharmaceuticals, © 2010Millennium Pharmaceuticals, Inc.

There were, at the time of this writing: Audit, National Marrow Donor Program, Santa Ana, CA, 2012; (714)800-1600.

Chapter 16

On an annual basis: K. Schulman, J. Kohles, "Economic Burden of Metastatic Bone Disease in the U.S.," published online April 20, 2007, Wiley InterScience, © American Cancer Society. R. Cook, "Economic and Clinical Impact of Multiple Myeloma to Managed Care," *Journal of Managed Care Pharmacy* 14, no.7 (2008): S18–S11.

Certainly, death panel *is too harsh:* National Commission on Fiscal Responsibility and Reform, "A Moment of Truth," Dec. 2010, endorses an Independent Payment Advisory Board, making it the ultimate arbiter of which treatments, and for what length of time, will be reimbursed through Medicare.

Similar thinking: "'Death Panels' Come Back to Life" David B. Rivkin, Jr., and Elizabeth Price Foley, *Wall Street Journal,* December 30, 2010: Congress's 2009 stimulus bill spent $1.1 billion to research "comparative effectiveness," the same approach used by Britain's National Health Service to weigh cost against factors including "quality of life." Also see mandate of Medicare's Independent Payment Advisory Board.

"This battleship has gone through wars": Los Angeles City Councilwoman Janice Hahn's comment was made to the *Los Angeles Times,* November 19, 2010, after several years of politicking. The *Iowa* finally made it

to Pier 93, San Pedro harbor district of L.A., two and a half years later.

Chapter 17

"Holistic spiritual practice and physical exercise": Cathy Eng, "Are Herbal Medicines Ripe for the Cancer Clinic?" *Science Translational Medicine Journal* 2, no.45 (August 18, 2010): 45ps41. Eng is with the Department of Gastrointestinal Medical Oncology, University of Texas, MD Anderson Cancer Center.

What You Need to Know About the FDA and Regulation: History in this section is from the FDA History Office, White Oak Building 31, room 3320, 10903 New Hampshire Avenue, Silver Spring, Maryland 30993.

Any natural product on the market: www.fda.gov/AboutFDA/whatwedo/history

As an example, if one takes oolong tea: By law, dietary supplements that were sold in the United States before 1964 may be marketed without evidence of efficacy or safety. Pieter A. Cohen, MD, "Assessing Supplement Safety," *New England Journal of Medicine* 366 (February 2, 2012): 389-391.

Meanwhile the FDA has received: Ibid.

A 2010 study sponsored by the National Cancer Institute: W. Lam, S. Bussom, F. Guan, et al., "The Four-Herb Chinese Medicine PHY906 Reduces Chemotherapy-Induced Gastrointestinal Toxicity," *Science Translational Medicine* 2, (2010): 45–59.

Chapter 18

Complementary Therapies: Particular thanks to Gary Deng, MD, PhD, Integrative Medicine Service, Memorial Sloan-Kettering Cancer Center, New York City, CME lecture, *Emerging Solutions in Pain,* 2012.

Although this method requires: http://www.livestrong.com/article/465013-exercises-for-the-mental-control-of-pain/#ixzz2AQ80ZF40

World Health Organization Guidelines: Controlling Pain, by Wendye R. Robbins, MD, and Ernest H. Rosenbaum, MD; *Everyone's Guide to Cancer Therapy,* (Kansas City, MO: Andrews McMeel Publishing, 2008), 202.

About the Authors

Jim Tamkin, MD, FACP, FACE, lived with myeloma for 11 years. He co-founded the TBA (Their Best Advice) Foundation with Dave Visel in 2009 to provide myeloma patients with the resources they need to cope with the disease. He worked as an internist and endocrinologist in Los Angeles until his death in March 2011.

Dave Visel is co-founder of the TBA Foundation and author of *Living with Cancer: A Practical Guide.* He is a retired advertising copywriter and marketing executive, and is a caregiver to his wife, Karen, who has lymphoma. They live in Los Angeles.

www.TBAfoundation.org

Back Cover Material

THE DEFINITIVE GUIDE TO LIVING A LONGER, FULLER LIFE WITH MYELOMA

The Myeloma Survival Guide makes sense of the difficult questions myeloma patients face, dealing with every aspect of life after diagnosis, from creating a wellness team to navigating treatment options to building a financial safety net. Jim Tamkin, MD, who lived with myeloma for 11 years, and Dave Visel share the insights they've gained as a doctor, patient, and caregiver, including:

- Everything you need to know about drugs and treatments, including stem cell transplants
- How to deal with the pain and side effects of chemotherapy, radiation, and surgery
- Insurance and tax benefits to save money and get you the care you deserve
- Take-charge tools you can use today to feel better tomorrows

"An invaluable guide to patients with newly diagnosed multiple myeloma. Not only have they provided clear information on the disease and its treatment, but most importantly also convey critical guidance on how to deal with the very personal life-impacting effects of this disease for patients and family members alike."

—**Kenneth C. Anderson,** MD, Kraft Family Professor of Medicine, Harvard Medical School, and Director, Jerome Lipper Multiple Myeloma Center and LeBow Institute for Myeloma Therapeutics, Dana-Farber Cancer Institute

***

Jim Tamkin, MD, FACP, FACE, lived with myeloma for 11 years. He co-founded the TBA (Their Best Advice) Foundation with Dave Visel in 2009 to provide myeloma patients with the resources they need to cope with the disease. He worked as an internist and endocrinologist in Los Angeles until his death in March 2011.

Dave Visel is co-founder of the TBA Foundation and author of *Living with Cancer: A Practical Guide.* He is a retired advertising copywriter and marketing executive, and is a caregiver to his wife, Karen, who has lymphoma. They live in Los Angeles.

WWW.TBAFOUNDATION.ORG

A

D

E

F

G

H

I

N

Q

R

S

T

U

V

W

Made in United States
Orlando, FL
04 November 2026

90202358R00203